Publisher's Note

R.G. Landes Company publishes six book series: *Medical Intelligence Unit, Molecular Biology Intelligence Unit, Neuroscience Intelligence Unit, Tissue Engineering Intelligence Unit, Environmental Intelligence Unit* and *Biotechnology Intelligence Unit.* The authors of our books are acknowledged leaders in their fields and the topics are unique. Almost without exception, no other similar books exist on these topics.

Our goal is to publish books in important and rapidly changing areas of medicine for sophisticated researchers and clinicians. To achieve this goal, we have accelerated our publishing program to conform to the fast pace in which information grows in biomedical science. Most of our books are published within 90 to 120 days of receipt of the manuscript. We would like to thank our readers for their continuing interest and welcome any comments or suggestions they may have for future books.

Deborah Muir Molsberry
Publications Director
R.G. Landes Company

BIOTECHNOLOGY INTELLIGENCE UNIT

STRUCTURE-PROPERTY CORRELATIONS IN DRUG RESEARCH

Han van de Waterbeemd, Ph.D.

F. Hoffmann-La Roche Ltd.
Pharma Research New Technologies
Basel, Switzerland

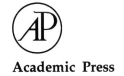

Academic Press

R.G. LANDES COMPANY
AUSTIN

BIOTECHNOLOGY INTELLIGENCE UNIT

STRUCTURE-PROPERTY CORRELATIONS IN DRUG RESEARCH

R.G. LANDES COMPANY
Austin, Texas, U.S.A.

Submitted: December 1995
Published: February 1996

This book is printed on acid-free paper.

Please address all inquiries to the Publisher:
R.G. Landes Company
909 Pine Street, Georgetown, Texas, U.S.A. 78626
Phone: 512/ 863 7762; FAX: 512/ 863 0081

Academic Press, Inc.
525 B Street, Suite 1900, San Diego, California, U.S.A. 92101-4495

United Kingdom Edition published by Academic Press Limited
24-28 Oval Road, London NW1 7DX, United Kingdom

International Standard Book Number (ISBN): ISBN 0-12-711650-8

Printed in the United States of America

While the authors, editors and publisher believe that drug selection and dosage and the specifications and usage of equipment and devices, as set forth in this book, are in accord with current recommendations and practice at the time of publication, they make no warranty, expressed or implied, with respect to material described in this book. In view of the ongoing research, equipment development, changes in governmental regulations and the rapid accumulation of information relating to the biomedical sciences, the reader is urged to carefully review and evaluate the information provided herein.

Library of Congress Cataloging-in-Publication Data

CIP INFORMATION APPLIED FOR BUT NOT YET RECEIVED.

CONTENTS

EDITOR

Han van de Waterbeemd, Ph.D.
F. Hoffmann-La Roche Ltd.
Pharma Research New Technologies
Basel, Switzerland
Chapters 1, 3

CONTRIBUTORS

Manfred Kansy, Ph.D.
F. Hoffmann-La Roche Ltd.
Pharma Research New Technologies
Basel, Switzerland
Chapter 2

David J. Livingstone, Ph.D.
ChemQuest, Cheyney House, Steeple Morden, Herts
The Centre for Molecular Design, University of Portsmouth,
Mercantile House, Portsmouth
United Kingdom
Chapter 4

C. John Blankley, Ph.D.
Parke-Davis Pharmaceutical Research
Ann Arbor, Michigan, U.S.A
Chapter 5

Michael S. Lajiness, Ph.D.
Pharmacia & Upjohn, Inc.
Computer Aided Drug Discovery
Kalamazoo, Michigan, U.S.A.
Chapter 6

PREFACE

The discovery and optimization of a chemical lead to a drug is a costly process. Therefore in today's preclinical drug research teamwork and the use of the most advanced techniques is a key to success. The in depth analysis of large amounts of biological and chemical data is important for establishing and understanding structure-activity relationships.

This book gives an overview of statistical chemometric methods used in drug discovery. We also discuss the kind of data which can be analyzed, particularly focussing on the physicochemical description of molecules, which is of great importance for the transport through biological barriers of crucial interest to orally bioavailable drugs.

The traditional field of application of chemometric methods is the field of quantitative structure-activity relationships (QSAR) developed by Corwin Hansch and colleagues some three decades ago. Currently structure-property correlations (SPC) of various kinds form an integral part of the drug discovery and optimization process. This is illustrated by a number of examples. Multivariate statistical or chemometrical approaches are used in newer fields such as three-dimensional quantitative approaches (3D-QSAR), 3D database searching and rational design of combinatorial libraries. This book deals with both these aspects. First, recent progress in the rapidly growing field of 3D-QSAR is presented. Finally, methods are discussed to analyze the diversity in large structure databases in relation to high throughput screening and combinatorial chemistry approaches and how the rational use of this information contributes to the drug discovery process.

Han van de Waterbeemd
Basel, September 1995

CHAPTER 1

DESIGN OF BIOACTIVE COMPOUNDS

Han van de Waterbeemd

New bioactive compounds can potentially be used as products such as a drug,[1] pesticide or herbicide,[2] fragrance or perfume.[3] To be useful, such compounds must be able to enter the target species, including humans, distribute favorably and finally reach in sufficient quantity the macromolecular active site, such as an enzyme or a receptor. The design of such new chemical entities (NCE) is a highly challenging task.

The classic way to discover bioactive compounds was to synthesize large series of derivatives, test these on relevant animal models, and select the most promising ones for (clinical) trials on humans. A first step to reduce particularly the large amounts of test animals was the systematic screening of compounds on enzyme preparations, in vitro cell cultures and isolated organs. A further step forward was the increasing use of computers for molecular modeling and quantitative structure-activity relationship studies in the design process.[4-6,18] Of course further important contributions to what is now called rational molecular design come from other disciplines including protein crystallography, bio-NMR, biochemistry and molecular biology.[7] The interplay between various disciplines can be seen in Figure 1.1. The field of medicinal chemistry traditionally consisting mainly of the synthesis and analysis of new compounds was broadened considerably. Medicinal chemistry is

Structure-Property Correlations in Drug Research, edited by Han van de Waterbeemd. © 1996 R.G. Landes Company.

today defined as "the science that deals with the discovery or design of new therapeutic chemicals and their development into useful medicines"[8] or "a chemistry-based discipline, also involving aspects of biological, medical and pharmaceutical sciences, which is concerned with the discovery, design, identification and preparation of biologically active compounds, the interpretation of their mode of interaction at the molecular level and the study of their metabolism."[9]

Besides the important question of how to make the compound, the question of which compound to make is even more demanding. The desired profile is a complex relationship between physicochemical properties of a molecule and their affinity and selectivity for certain macromolecules, as well as the absorption, biotransformation and elimination profiles. The chances for successful design are largest when much relevant information can be taken into account. The level of understanding of what to do next largely is a function of the status of a project. In an early phase of a project this information may still be lacking. In this exploratory phase a wide sampling of property space should be taken into consideration. This is mostly done by systematic variation of selected parts of a lead compound. A typical situation is the variation of a substituent, which can be done using tabulated properties of such substituent. As described in more detail in chapter 2, some descriptors are unique and just describe one feature, while others are composed. A prominent example is the much used partition coefficient in octanol/water (log P values). This property in fact is composed of a term related to the size of the molecule and to its hydrogen bonding capability.[12,13] Some descriptors may be called fuzzy parameters, since they are e.g. conformation-dependent, making their value variable within a certain range. In Table 1.1 an overview is given of different types of descriptors.

Increasingly time pressure on drug discovery projects forces parallel approaches in drug discovery. A comparison of a sequential and parallel drug discovery approach is presented in Figures 1.2 and 1.3. Nevertheless, the playground for the design of new compounds is limited (Fig. 1.4). On one side the compounds should not be too complicated, while on the other side they should be diverse and sample well the potential property space. At the same

Table 1.1. Types of molecular and substituent descriptors for use in SPC studies and library design

fuzzy / precise

global / local (molecular / substructural = fragmental)

composite / unique

experimental / calculated

2D (topological) / 3D (geometrical)

topological (e.g. lipophilic region) / functional (H-bond, charge)

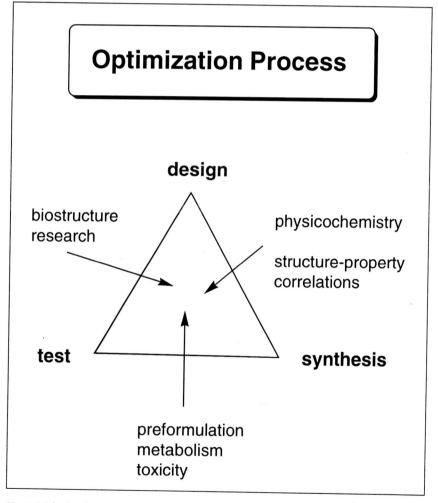

Fig. 1.1. The lead optimization process. The classical approach involved mainly the cycle design, synthesis and testing. Today these basic drug discovery functions get considerable support from other disciplines: biostructure research (crystallography, NMR, molecular modeling), physicochemistry and structure-property correlations, and the early involvement of the pharmacokinetics and formulation functions. New compounds increasingly come from combinatorial synthesis approaches.

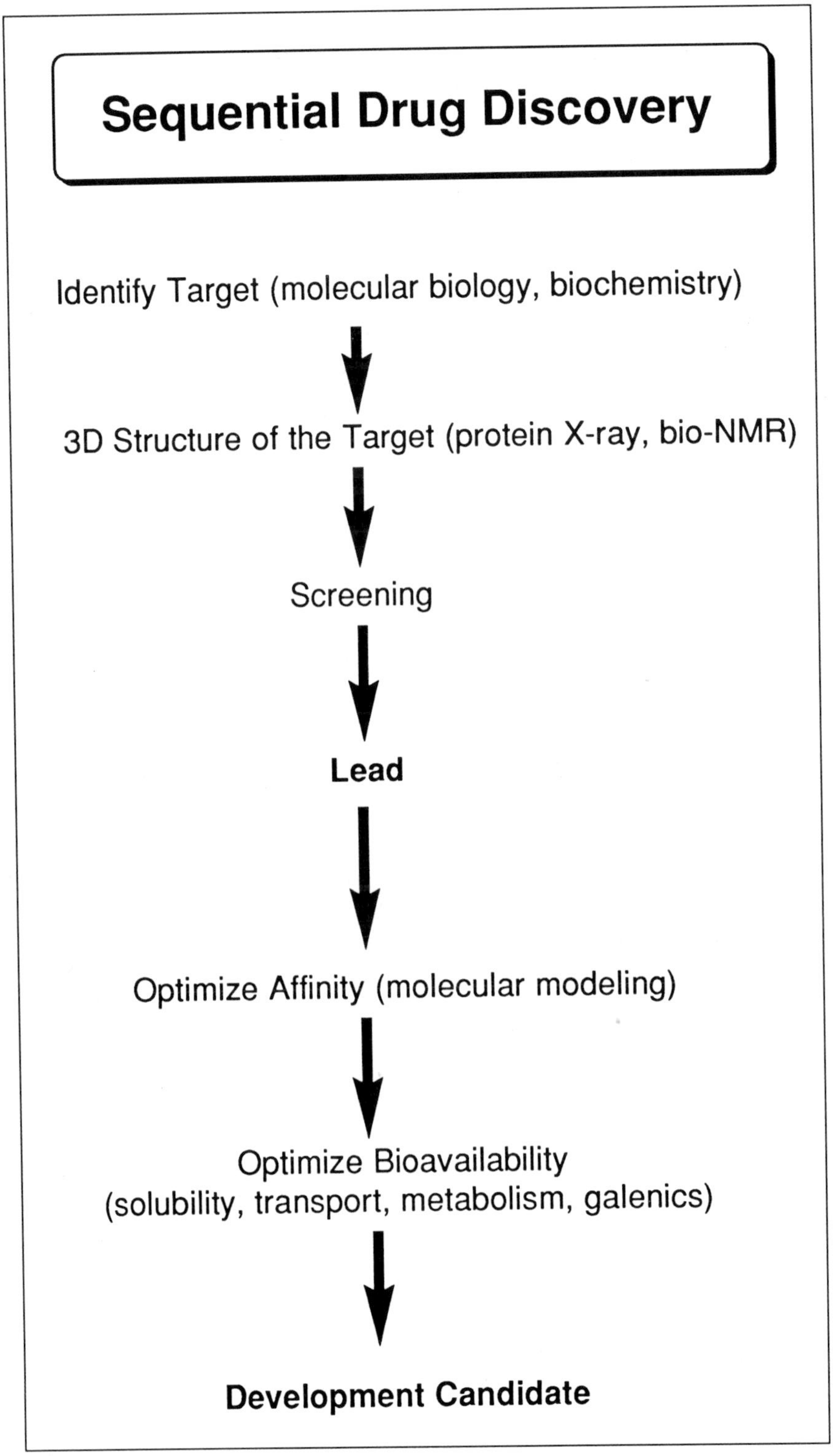

Sequential Drug Discovery

Identify Target (molecular biology, biochemistry)

↓

3D Structure of the Target (protein X-ray, bio-NMR)

↓

Screening

↓

Lead

↓

Optimize Affinity (molecular modeling)

↓

Optimize Bioavailability
(solubility, transport, metabolism, galenics)

↓

Development Candidate

Fig. 1.2. Traditional drug discovery was a sequential process. Shown here is the case where the macromolecular target has been identified and its three-dimensional structure resolved (design of enzyme inhibitors). In other cases leads may be found directly from screening.

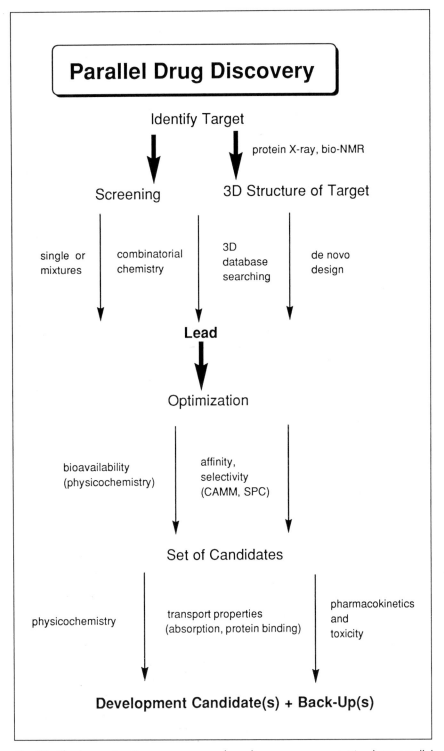

Fig. 1.3. *The increasing time pressure on drug discovery programs stimulates parallel approaches in drug discovery. CAMM = Computer-Assisted Molecular Modeling; SPC = Structure-Property Correlations.*

time there may be some other limitations. These may be structural (if structural information of the target is known) and/or physicochemical (solubility, lipophilicity) related to absorption and bioavailability of the desired compound. All these aspects make modern medicinal chemistry highly demanding.[10]

Structure-property correlation (SPC) studies are of interest to unravel the information in biological data from several tests, to look for potential correlations between biological and (physico) chemical data, and in the prediction of biophysical and physicochemical properties.[11] Molecular properties can be divided in three groups: intrinsic, chemical and biological (Fig. 1.5). Relationships

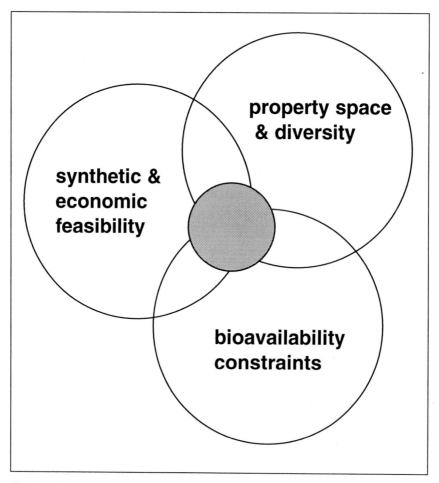

Fig. 1.4. Limitations in molecular design. A compromise must be made between synthetic/economic, molecular diversity and bioavailability aspects.

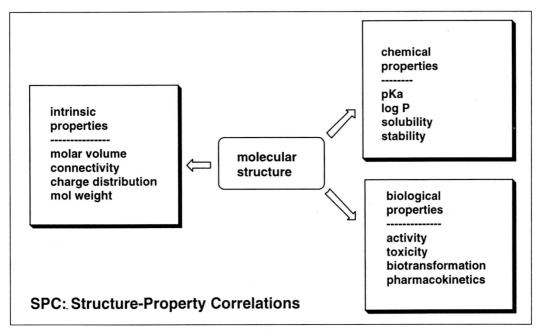

Fig. 1.5. The concept of structure-property correlations (SPC). Molecular properties can be defined on three levels, intrinsic, chemical and biological. Correlations among any of these may be of interest. When biological activities are involved, this may be referred to as quantitative structure-activity relationships (QSAR) or quantitative structure-toxicity relationships (QSTR), while the prediction of physical properties is called quantitative structure-property relationships (QSPR).[11] Data are reproduced with permission from Van de Waterbeemd H. Quant Struct-Act Relat 1992; 11:200-204.

may exist between any of these, in any combination. Chemometric methods based on statistical and mathematical approaches can be used to unravel putative relationships.

An important area of research is the description of molecular properties and the comparison among compounds.

The following chapters discuss different aspects of structure-property relationships. Therefore, first an overview is given of the most relevant properties and how these can be estimated, either experimentally or by computational approaches. Modern statistical approaches used to establish quantitative relationships between different kind of properties (e.g. biological and chemical), illustrated with several examples form the second part of the book. Next we summarize the progress made in the field of three-dimensional quantitative structure-activity relationships (3D-QSAR).[14] This technique is linking statistical approaches to molecular modeling[15] and had much attention over the last few years.[14] Finally, the last chapter deals with the description of molecular diversity and similarity.[16,17] This topic is increasingly important in the rational design of combinatorial libraries and the clustering of large databases for the selection of compounds for screening.

REFERENCES

1. Wolff ME, ed. Burger's Medicinal Chemistry and Drug Discovery. New York: Wiley, 1995.
2. Magee PS, Henry DR, Block JH, eds. Probing Bioactive Mechanisms. ACS Symposium Series 413. Washington: ACS, 1989.
3. Müller PM, Lamparsky D, eds. Perfumes. Art, Science and Technology. London: Elsevier, 1991.
4. Van de Waterbeemd H. The history of drug research: from Hansch to the present. Quant Struct-Act Relat 1992; 11:200-204.
5. Van de Waterbeemd H. Recent progress in QSAR-technology. Drug Des Discov 1993; 9:277-285.
6. Herrmann EC, Franke R. Computer Aided Drug Design in Industrial Research. Berlin: Springer, 1995.
7. Wermuth CG, Koga N, König H, Metcalf BW. Medicinal Chemistry for the 21st Century. Oxford: Blackwell, 1992.
8. Silverman RB. The Organic Chemistry of Drug Design and Drug Action. San Diego: Academic Press, 1992.
9. Wermuth CG, Ganellin CR, Imhof R et al. Glossary of terms used in medicinal chemistry. Recommendations 1995.
10. Wermuth CG, ed. The Practice of Medicinal Chemistry. London: Academic Press, 1995.
11. Murugan R, Grendze MP, Toomey JE Jr et al. Predicting physical properties from molecular structure. Chemtech 1994; 17-23.
12. van de Waterbeemd H, Testa B. The parametrization of lipophilicity and other structural properties in drug design. Adv Drug Res 1987; 16: 85-225.
13. El Tayar N, Testa B, Carrupt PA. Polar intermolecular interactions encoded in partition coefficients: an indirect estimation of hydrogen-bond parameters of polyfunctional solutes. J Phys Chem 1992; 96: 1456-1459.
14. Kubinyi H, ed. 3D QSAR in Drug Design. Theory, Methods and Applications. Leiden: ESCOM, 1993.
15. Vinter JG, Gardner M, eds. Molecular Modeling and Drug Design. London: Macmillan, 1994.
16. Johnson MA, Maggiora GM, eds. Concepts and Applications of Molecular Similarity. New York: John Wiley, 1990.

17. Dean PM, ed. Molecular Similarity in Drug Design. London: Chapman & Hall, 1995.
18. Dean PM, Jolles G, Newton CG, eds. New Perspectives in Drug Design. London: Academic Press, 1995.

MOLECULAR PROPERTIES

Manfred Kansy

INTRODUCTION

A significant reduction in time and costs for the overall drug discovery and optimization process is of major concern in preclinical research and development. In 1978 Seydel and Schaper[1] reported an average number of about 5000 compounds that had to be synthesized to get one drug on the market, but with combinatorial chemistry in place, the number of synthesized compounds is no longer an appropriate measure for the judgment of the efficiency of the drug discovery and development process. Calculated and experimental molecular properties have been influencing the different phases of the drug discovery and development process since the 1970s. However, do molecular properties have the same importance today, after nearly 25 years of progress in pharmaceutical research? What are the impacts of molecular and physicochemical properties on drug discovery and development today? Which properties are predominantly used in pharmaceutical research and how are these obtained? How will this field develop in the future?

Both the quantitative and qualitative relationships between structure and activity are important elements in pharmaceutical research. However, the earlier methods of quantitative structure-activity relationships (QSAR) are being supplemented by new ones. Computer-assisted molecular modeling (CAMM) including x-ray crystallography of the biological targets are providing the basis for

Structure-Property Correlations in Drug Research, edited by
Han van de Waterbeemd. © 1996 R.G. Landes Company.

more sophisticated techniques such as 3D-QSAR (see chapter 5). These methods allow more precise definitions of factors responsible for activity of compounds to be given on a structural basis, and thus provide an improved conceptual framework for the incorporation of experimental or calculated properties, as described in the following.

Terms like quantitative structure property relationships (QSPR), structure-property relationships (SPR) or structure-property correlations (SPC) have been introduced which reflect a paradigm shift in using molecular properties and structural information, becoming increasingly important in the description of properties relating to specific aspects of in vivo bioavailability, such as, for example, transport phenomena through biological barriers.

Combinatorial chemistry[2] has provided a new momentum to the field of molecular property evaluation and structure correlation. Thousands if not millions of compounds can be produced in a few synthetic steps using a set of chemical building blocks with all possible combinations. This will rapidly expand the stock of compounds, available for "high throughput screening" (HTS) in most of the major pharmaceutical companies. However, reduction of possible redundancy by avoiding the synthesis of many similar end products is one key issue in this area. Clearly, in a combinatorial synthesis program it may not be necessary to use all possible combinations of building blocks which are commercially available. In order to overcome the combinatorial explosion the challenge consists in defining minimal combinations with maximum diversity, resulting in the need to assess the diversity/similarity of the used building blocks and the resulting end products. Diversity can be described by a number of different physicochemical or calculated properties.[2] In principle all properties used in the traditional field of SAR are usable in the diversity planning in combinatorial chemistry. Experimental values often do not exist for the large number of building blocks, and calculated properties have to be used instead. The number of available relevant properties is rather restricted, since many commonly used properties are often interrelated.

Applications of 3D-database searching represents another area where considerations of molecular properties are becoming increasingly important[3-6] (see chapter 6). A major challenge in this field is the reduction of the chemical structural information to a few relevant property descriptors oriented in 3D-space. In 3D-database searching normally pharmacophore models[7] derived from knowledge of target structures, biomechanistic aspects or active compounds are used. In order to reduce search times, the spatial orientation of the major fragment properties of a compound are stored, making 3D-database searches including larger numbers of possible conformations very fast.

Transport processes through biological barriers, viz., the passive diffusion through biological membranes is another area where structure-property correlations are of interest. Although potency and selectivity are key issues in drug discovery, other factors like solubility, absorption, partitioning or biodegradation are equally important. Unfortunately, optimization with regard to these properties often sets in at later stages in the overall discovery/development process and may therefore negatively impact on the chemical program by forcing late shifts of focus with concomitant delays. An early assessment of molecular properties may avoid such problems by assisting the lead optimization process with relevant data. For example it is well known that the pK_a and the lipophilicity of a compound, which is expressed by the distribution coefficient log D, strongly influence its absorption.[8] Likewise, the solubility and dissolution rate of a compound influence absorption. Furthermore the size of a compound, often expressed by its molecular weight, is a further measure often used in the mathematical description of transport processes.

In the following essential molecular properties which are currently used in pharmaceutical research are described. Good correlations between calculated and experimental values are often found in the literature. However, this does not imply that the calculation methods are infallible. Therefore, after a short excursion into the field of tabulated and structure-derived properties, the following chapters emphasize the experimental methods and physicochemical properties used in the contexts of the drug discovery and development process. Possible calculation methods for these properties will be mentioned.

Table 2.1. Selection of tabulated and structure-derived molecular properties

- Polarizability parameters, e.g. molar refractivity (MR).

- Electronic parameters, e.g. Hammett σ constants, field $\mathfrak{I}$ and resonance parameters $\mathfrak{R}$, dipole moments, charge transfer constants.
- Steric parameters, e.g. E_s, E_s^c, v, and the STERIMOL parameters B_1 to B_5 and L.

- Topological parameters, e.g. connectivity indices.

- Hydrogen bonding parameters, and values derived from quantum chemical calculations.

- Molecular surface and volume.

- Others, e.g. molecular weight, indicator variables.

CALCULATED AND TABULATED PROPERTIES

SUBSTITUENT CONSTANTS

Recently a large number of reviews[9-15] on molecular properties were published, focusing on the classical descriptors used in QSAR studies. In principle these parameters can be subdivided as depicted in Table 2.1. For a complete overview on these parameters we refer to these reviews.

Since 1995[16] a revision of the parameters collected and published earlier by Leo and Hansch in 1979 is available, including π, σ, MR, $\mathfrak{I}$, $\mathfrak{R}$ parameter values for more than 3000 different substituents. A general overview on more than 200 parameters has been given by van de Waterbeemd and Testa.[17] This table has been extended by additional parameters and is included in commercially available databases and QSAR tools like the TSAR[18] software.

Extensive statistical studies have been performed in attempts to extract the principal properties from the large number of currently used molecular descriptors. The information content like the one contained in Table 2.1 can be reduced to few dimensions by multivariate statistical methods such as principal component (PCA)[19] or factor analyses (FA).[19] Variables which are highly interrelated are grouped into factors or principal components (PC) which are orthogonal to each other. The principal components are correlated with biological activity values in a further independent step. By contrast to PCA, the partial least squares method (PLS) works with vectors for both, structural descriptors and biological activities, which are extracted simultaneously. PLS[20-22] is particularly suited for problems where large numbers of descriptors are used to rationalize comparatively small numbers of observations. Various studies on substituent data sets have been performed using these techniques. A set of 40 variables has been examined using PCA analysis.[25] Eight so-called disjoint principal properties (DPPs) have been extracted. DPPs, in contrast to PCs are not mutually orthogonal. They can be used in partial least square analysis, but not in multiple linear regression studies.

Multidimensional scaling (MDS)[23,24] is a method for data reduction, usable on similarity and dissimilarity matrices. It has been applied in the reduction of the number of possible building blocks in combinatorial chemistry.[2]

Kubinyi[26,27] describes an interesting approach for variable selection using an evolutionary algorithm.

STRUCTURE-DERIVED PROPERTIES

Besides the tabulated properties, descriptors can be derived directly from a structure. Although these properties are easily obtained by different computer programs and therefore often used, their usefulness may be questioned.

Topological descriptors are derived directly from the graph of a structure. The most widely used topological descriptors are the ones introduced by Kier and Hall.[28,29] Although such descriptors have been used for the description of various structural properties, their meaning and value remains unclear. Recently Kier and Hall[31] have introduced some new so-called atom-level descriptors,[30,31] which have been used in QSAR studies.[32] Whether these new descriptors offer advantages in comparison to topological indices remains to be seen. Kubinyi[33] gives a brief, but excellent overview on the relevance of currently available topological indices as well as their use and misuse.

Hydrogen bonding is an important factor for ligand binding. The H-bonding capacity has been extensively studied in the identification of the physicochemical properties governing solubility and partitioning phenomena.[34] Although the strengths of hydrogen bonds in principle can be calculated using dipole moments of the interacting groups or partial charges,[35] tabulated parameters describing the strengths of hydrogen bonds are limited to a few sources.[13] Abraham and coworkers[36,37] measured proton donor and acceptor properties for more than 150 compounds in a standard-

Table 2.2. Collection of aromatic substituent constants

Substituent	Lipophilic		Steric		Electronic			
	π_{ar}	π_{al}	E_s	E_s^c	σ	σ^*	$\Im$	$\Re$
BROMO	0.86	0.6	-0.08	0.84	0.083	0.122	0.44	-0.17
CHLORO	0.71	0.39	-0.27	0.65	0.068	0.099	0.41	-0.15
FLUORO	0.14	-0.17	-0.78	0.14	0.051	0.078	0.43	-0.34
IODO	1.12	1	0.16	1.08	0.095	0.133	0.4	-0.19
NITRO	-0.28	-0.85	0.28	2.2	0.13	0.17	0.67	0.16
HYDROGEN	0	0	-1.24	-0.32	0	0	0	0
HYDROXYL	-0.67	-1.12	-0.69	-0.08	0.067	0.11	0.29	-0.64
THIOL	0.39	0.28	-0.17	0.44	0.097	0.137	0.28	-0.11
AMINO	-1.23	-1.19	-0.63	-0.32	0.075	0.115	0.02	-0.68
SULPHAMOYL	-1.82	-1.71	0.41	1.3	0.145	0.18	0.41	0.19
TRIFLUOROMETHYL	0.88	0.29	1.16	2.08	0.142	0.187	0.38	0.19
TRIFLUOROMETHOXY	1.04	0.41	0.44	0.65	0.145	0.18	0.38	0
TRIFLUOROMETHANE SULPHONYL	0.55	0.07	1	1.45	0.2	0.25	0.73	0.26
TRIFLUOROMETHYLTHIO	1.44	0.71	0.5	1.07	0.16	0.2	0.35	0.18
CYANO	-0.57	-0.84	-0.73	0.19	0.077	0.12	0.51	0.19
ISOTHIOCYANATO	0.41	0.03	0.14	0.9	0.13	0.165	0.36	0.19
THIOCYANATO	1.15	0.49	0.14	0.69	0.13	0.165	0.51	-0.09
FORMYL	-0.65	-0.84	-0.23	0.62	0.127	0.152	0.31	0.13
CARBOXY	-0.32	-0.67	-0.23	0.62	0.1	0.13	0.33	0.15
CARBAMOYL	-1.49	-1.71	-0.23	0.51	0.11	0.135	0.24	0.14
OCONH2	-1.05	-1.17	0.25	0.57	0.135	0.17	0.15	0.1
METHYL	0.56	0.5	0	0	0.076	0.091	-0.04	-0.13
METHOXYL	-0.02	-0.37	-0.69	0.23	0.127	0.156	0.26	-0.51
HYDROXYMETHYL	-1.03	-1.12	-0.03	0.28	0.09	0.11	0	0
UREIDO	-1.3	-1.26	0.3	0.6	0.135	0.17	0.04	-0.28
METHANESULPHONYL	-1.63	-1.5	0.5	1.45	0.18	0.232	0.54	0.22
METHANETHIO	0.61	0.09	-0.17	0.75	0.15	0.186	0.2	-0.18
METHYLAMINO	-0.47	-0.67	-0.58	0.18	0.09	0.115	-0.11	-0.74
ACETYLENYL	0.4	0.48	-0.03	0.7	0.09	0.11	0.19	0.05
CYANOMETHYL	-0.57	-0.86	1.14	1.45	0.11	0.14	0.21	-0.18
VINYL	0.82	0.19	-0.26	0.6	0.09	0.11	0.07	-0.08
ACETYL	-0.55	-0.62	0.05	0.75	0.141	0.2	0.32	0.2
METHOXYCARBONYL	-0.01	-0.3	0.36	0.94	0.2	0.254	0.33	0.15
ACETOXY	-0.64	-0.27	-0.23	0.35	0.135	0.17	0.41	-0.07
CH2COOH	-0.72	-0.86	0.37	0.8	0.14	0.175	0.15	0.1
OCH2COOH	-0.79	-0.95	0.23	0.55	0.125	0.16	0.15	0.05
ACETAMIDO	-0.97	-1.03	0.4	0.6	0.145	0.18	0.28	-0.26

ized format to lay the basis for a database system. The number of existing H-bond donor and acceptor sites in a molecule were used as descriptors for the H-bonding capacity and corresponding tabulated parameter values exist.[38] Recently, an interesting approach has been described relating H-bonding capacities to experimental log P values and molar volumes.[39]

Table 2.2. Collection of aromatic substituent constants (continued)

Substituent	Lipophilic		Steric		Electronic			
	π_{ar}	π_{al}	E_s	E_s^c	σ	σ^*	$\Im$	$\Re$
METHOXYCARBONYL								
AMINO	-0.37	-0.6	0.65	0.8	0.165	0.21	0.14	-0.28
ETHYL	1.02	0.41	0.07	0.38	0.127	0.161	-0.05	-0.1
ETHOXY	0.38	0.03	-0.29	0.32	0.12	0.15	0.22	-0.44
DIMETHYLAMINO	0.18	-0.3	-0.45	0	0.134	0.191	0.1	-0.92
CYCLOPROPYL	1.14	0.51	1.58	1.35	0.12	0.145	-0.03	-0.19
ETHOXYCARBONYL	0.51	0.07	0.44	0.98	0.155	0.195	0.33	0.15
PROPYL	1.55	0.8	0.36	0.67	0.125	0.155	-0.06	-0.08
ISOPROPYL	1.53	0.79	0.47	1.08	0.159	0.199	-0.05	-0.1
PROPOXY	1.05	0.45	-0.03	0.45	0.135	0.17	0.22	-0.45
ISOPROPOXY	0.36	0.45	0.58	0.7	0.15	0.19	0.3	-0.72
BUTYL	2.13	1.22	0.39	0.7	0.16	0.2	-0.06	-0.11
TERT-BUTYL	1.98	1.17	1.54	2.48	0.173	0.21	-0.07	-0.13
BUTYLOXY	1.55	1.03	0.03	0.45	0.145	0.18	0.25	-0.55
BUTYLAMINO	1.45	0.68	0.42	0.65	0.155	0.19	-0.28	-0.25
DIETHYLAMINO	1.18	0.57	2.58	2.5	0.19	0.235	0.01	-0.91
PENTYL	2.67	1.62	0.4	0.71	0.145	0.18	-0.06	-0.08
PHENYL	1.96	2.15	2.55	2	0.164	0.236	0.08	-0.08
PHENOXY	2.08	0.47	0.75	0.75	0.165	0.21	0.34	-0.35
ANILINO	1.37	0.2	0.8	0.75	0.17	0.215	-0.02	-0.38
CYCLOHEXYL	2.51	1.62	0.79	1.4	0.16	0.2	-0.13	-0.1
BENZOYL	1.05	0.36	1	1.25	0.2	0.245	0.3	0.16
CH2CH2C6H5	2.66	1.65	0.38	0.69	0.165	0.21	-0.03	-0.01

π_{ar}: Aromatic hydrophobic fragment constant.

π_{al}: Aliphatic hydrophobic fragment constant.

E_s: Taft steric parameter.

E_s^c: corrected Taft steric parameter (considering effect of hydrogens on α carbon).

σ: Hamett constant.

σ^*: Inductive polar constant from Taft.

$\Im$: Field parameter.

$\Re$: Resonance parameter.

(Reproduced with permission from: van de Waterbeemd H, Testa B. The parametirization of lipophilicity and other structural properties in drug research. Adv Drug Res 1987; 16:85-225.)

Dipole moments (μ) for 300 compounds have been compiled by Lien and coworkers[40] and compared with polar substituent constants σ^* and the electronic substituent constant σ.[41] Using dipole moments, good correlations were obtained for the description of bioactivities of anticonvulsants and anti-depressants.[42] The role of dipole moments in ligand receptor interaction has been further discussed by Oprea.[43]

Molecular surfaces and volumes can be calculated from the 3D-coordinates of molecular structures, using well-known methods.[44-46] It has been shown that these properties can be used in the description of partition phenomena,[44,48] solubility[47] or transport through membranes.[39]

Besides lipophilicity and the ionization constant (pK_a), the molecular weight (MW) may serve as a parameter in the description of permeation processes.[49,50] Like the volume term, MW negatively influences permeation processes when the size is becoming the limiting step in transport.[50] Examination of the different drug databases with respect to molecular weights reveals that most drugs have MW between 300-400 (Fig. 2.2),[51] a MW-range where transport should be little influenced by size. Although MW can be easily calculated, its replacement by a structure-derived size descriptor would be desirable.

The use of quantum chemical (QC) descriptors for biological problems has been reviewed by Thomson.[52] A large number of QC-descriptors[53-55] are available and have been used in SAR studies.[56] Tabulated charges or methods for rapid calculations[57,58] of charge distributions in molecules have been used in these studies.

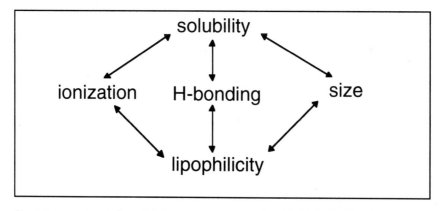

Fig. 2.1. Properties influencing transport processes through biological barriers.

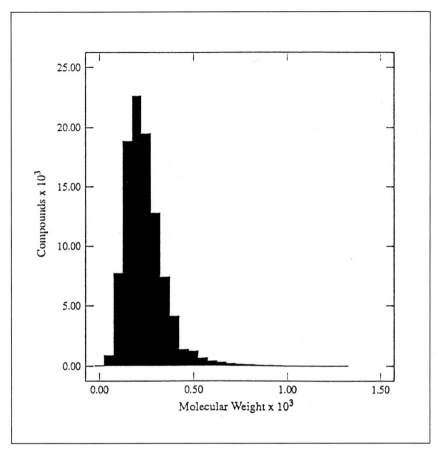

Fig. 2.2. Typical molecular weight distribution in a drug database. X-axis: molecular weight; Y-axis: Number of compounds (with permision of CATALYST V2.3. Molecular Simulations).

The application of atomic charge distributions with an extended parameter set in SAR analysis has been discussed by Dixon and Jurs.[59]

Indicator variables or dummy variables can be used to signal the existence of a structural fragment in a specific position of a compound where otherwise no descriptor values are available, thus significantly extending the application range of QSAR studies (Free Wilson analysis[60]).

PHYSICOCHEMICAL PROPERTIES: MEASUREMENT AND PREDICTION

LIPOPHILICITY

Lipophilicity describes the partitioning of a solute between an aqueous and an organic solvent, e.g., 1-octanol.

$$P = \frac{{}^{c}\text{organic phase}}{{}^{c}\text{aqueous phase}} \tag{1}$$

Although the use of 1-octanol has major advantages because of its donor and acceptor properties,[10] the 1-octanol/water system as a standard has been questioned.

Statistical analyses of partition coefficients for different solvents have shown that lipophilicities described by log P_{oct} values depend on the solute bulk and hydrogen bonding effects.[61,62] Partition coefficients for phospholipid-micelle/water systems can differ dramatically from those observed in 1-octanol/water.[63-70] This indicates, that 1-octanol/water may not be an appropriate system for the description of the partition processes in membranes. Indeed, the problems associated with log P_{oct} values for the description of transport processes may arise from the hydrogen bond donor and acceptor properties of 1-octanol. These are different from those of the constituents of biological membranes like for example phospholipids. However, through the large number of partition coefficients determined for the 1-octanol/water system the log P_{oct} has become a de facto standard in the description of partition phenomena in drug research and toxicology. In the meantime, an increasing number of other organic solvent systems[71] have been used for the determination of partition coefficients. For example propylene glycol dipelargonate (PGDP) has been suggested as an additional solvent for partition studies.[72]

The relation between partition coefficients determined in different solvents is described by the Collander Equation[73] in a linear relationship.

$$\log P_{\text{solvent 1}} = a \log P_{\text{solvent2}} + b \tag{2}$$

$$\Delta\log P = \log P_{\text{solvent 1}} - \log P_{\text{solvent2}} \tag{3}$$

Seiler[74,75] was one of the first in defining the hydrogen bonding ability I_h of a set of functional groups, by measuring the log P values in different organic solvent/water systems. The Δlog P value (Equation 3) has been introduced in the description of transport processes, especially in the transport through the blood/brain barrier.[76,77] Unfortunately two time-consuming measurements are necessary for the determination of a Δlog P value. Testa and Seiler[78] could show that log P_{oct} is a composite parameter (Equation 4), consisting of a cavity and a polarity term, where V is the van der Waals volume and Λ describes polarity including H-bonding capacity. The values derived from measurements of log P_{oct} were observed to correlate with the H-bond acceptor basicity (β), while those derived from partition studies in alkane/water mixtures relate to total H-bond capacities.[79]

$$\log P = aV - \Lambda \tag{4}$$

Using calculated hydrophilic surfaces of a solute and a molecular volume descriptor, penetration processes through the blood/brain barrier can be described.[77] Furthermore, molecular volumes can be easily used in the calculation of Λ values if log P_{oct} values are known.

Paterson et al[80] uses another approach for the rationalization of transport processes through membranes. They avoid the time-consuming determination of Δlog P values by introducing the heptane/glycol partitioning system. The observed partition coefficients in this solvent system show a good correlation with permeability coefficients through Caco-2 cell monolayers,[81] a cell culture system used in the estimation of cell penetration of drugs.

MEASUREMENT OF LIPOPHILICITY PROPERTIES

The determination of partition coefficients or related parameters is not an easy task. Several methods are known for the determination of partition coefficients.[82] Besides the well-known shake flask method, the standard procedure for log P_{oct} determinations, several new methods have been introduced. Centrifugal partition chromatography (CPC)[83-89] is an automated liquid/liquid system using centrifugal forces for the separation of the two solvent phases. El Tayar and Tsai[83,84] described this technique for different solvent systems. This technique allows a fast log P_{oct} determination in the range -3 < log P_{oct} < 3. In principle log P values of mixtures can be determined by CPC. Unfortunately, instruments available on the market are still not sufficiently robust. Recently Livingstone[90] introduced another method for the determination of partition coefficients of mixtures.

Table 2.3. Comparison of correction functions used in log P_{oct} or log k'_w determinations

pK$_a$ correction functions	
Simplified logarithmic	**Empirical**
monoprotic acids: $\log k_0 = \log k + \log(1+10^{pH-pK_a})$	$\log k_0 = \log k + (1-\tanh(pK_a-pH+1))$
monoprotic bases: $\log k_0 = \log k + \log(1+10^{pK_a-pH})$	$\log k_0 = \log k + (1-\tanh(pH-pK_a+1))$
diprotic acids and bases: $\log k_0 = \log k + \log(1+10^{pH-pK_{a1}}+10^{2pH-pK_{a1}-pK_{a2}})$ $\log k_0 = \log k + \log(1+10^{pK_{a1}-pH}+10_{pKa1+pKa2-2pH})$	for pK$_{aacid} \leq 5$ at a pH of 7.4 $\log k_0 = \log k + 2$

k_0: pK$_a$-corrected log k'$_w$ (log k) (equivalent shake flask: P)
k'$_w \equiv$ log k: not pK$_a$-corrected (equivalent shake flask: D)

A filterprobe/filter chamber method has been introduced by Hersey et al.[91] The method is again more comfortable than the shake flask method. The system consists of a chamber separated by a filter paper from a compartment connected to a photometer, thus avoiding 1-octanol entering the measuring cell. pH-dependent log D determinations are possible with the filterprobe/filter chamber method. However, this method again is limited to a range of -3 < log P$_{oct}$ < 3 as is true for the CPC method and has the disadvantage to be usable only for pure compounds. If a compound contains ionizable groups, the measurement range can be enhanced by the determination of the distribution coefficient of the ionized species (log D) by choosing a suitable pH of the buffer. The log P$_{oct}$ value can be easily calculated from the measured log D values by well-known equations (Table 2.3).

The potentiometric measurement in organic solvent/water systems represents another important method for the determination of log P$_{oct}$ and log D, if the compound of interest contains ionizable groups. This method allows distribution profiles of very lipophilic compounds to be measured up to log P$_{oct}$ values of ca. 7.[92]

The pK_a of the compound has to be known or determined in a first run. The method, first described by Brandström,[93] Seiler[75] and Clarke[94,95] has been modified and substantially improved by Avdeef and coworkers.[96-99] Including the measurement of pK_a in organic solvent/water mixtures, distribution coefficients in organic solvent/water or micelle/water systems, the potentiometric measurement is fast and gives excellent results. For a log D determination the difference in the pK_a and apparent pK_a according to Equation 5 are used, where r is the ratio between organic and aqueous solvents and p_oK_a is the apparent pK_a in the titration with 1-octanol.

$$P = \frac{10^{p_oK_a - pK_a} - 1}{r} \tag{5}$$

Other approaches to liquid/liquid partition systems make use of high-performance liquid chromatography (HPLC) and thin-layer chromatography (TLC),[100] providing fast and virtually unrestricted methods for the determination of lipophilicity properties of compounds.[101-107] The advantages of these methods lie in the fact that small amounts of compound are required and that compounds do not have to be pure. Water insoluble compounds can be measured, since organic solvent/buffer mixtures are generally chosen as mobile phase. The measure for the lipophilicity in this system is the log k' value calculated from the retention time of the solute (t_r) and the dead time (t_0) of a non-retained compound.

$$\log k' = \log(t_r - t_0)/t_0 \tag{6}$$

The log k'_w value is the result of an extrapolation of a series log k' determinations derived by measurements under different organic modifier/buffer mixtures as depicted in Figure 2.3.[108,109] The advantage of the linear extrapolation over the non-linear extrapolation method is discussed by Testa,[110] also in cases where a non-linear relation between modifier content and log k' is observed. Often this non-linear behavior between organic modifier content and log k' is seen when ionized compounds are measured and organic solvents with a low dipole moment are used (Fig. 2.4). Different column types are described in the determination of lipophilic descriptors by HPLC. Unger[111] was one of the first to describe the measurement of retention times on octanol-coated

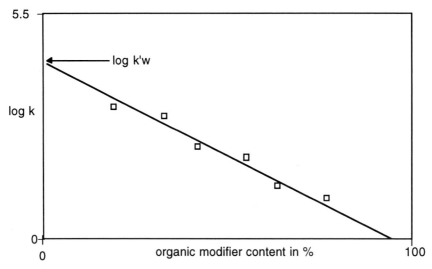

Fig. 2.3. Linear extrapolation using measured log k' values obtained at different organic modifier/buffer ratios for the determination of the log k'$_w$ -value.

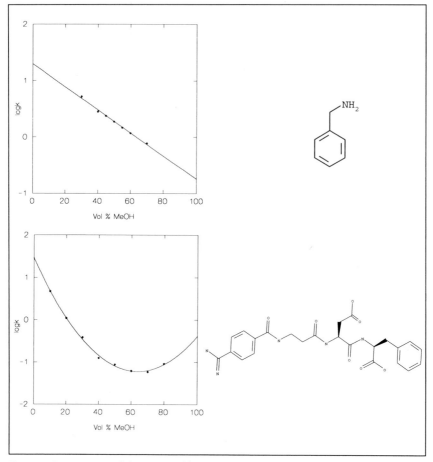

Fig. 2.4. Comparison of the extrapolation methods on two test examples. Non-linear: RO-43-5054 (pH 7.4); linear: benzylamin (pH 7.4)

reversed-phase (RP) HPLC columns, showing good correlations with known $\log P_{oct}$ values. Problems may arise from octanol bubbles in the mobile phase disturbing the detector signal.

Beside the well-known reversed-phase octadecyl silanol (ODS) columns, octadecyl polyvinyl (ODP) polymer columns have shown advantages in the measurement of lipophilicity properties.[112,113] One major advantage of polymer columns is the avoidance of the solute interaction with free silanol groups.

IAM (immobilized artificial membrane) columns[114-118] have been introduced recently. Solutes can show a totally different behavior on this column type through an additional ionic interaction with the phospholipid head groups of the column. Retention times observed by measurements on this column gave slightly better correlations with membrane permeability than $\log k'$ values determined on common RP-columns, especially when a size descriptor like the molecular weight was additionally considered.

For ionizable compounds a correlation of $\log k'_w$-values with $\log P_{oct}$ values requires a correction for the ionization states of the compounds. In case of a direct correlation of $\log k'_w$ with $\log P_{oct}$ a correction to the neutral species is necessary. Several equations have been described to correct $\log k'_w$-values.[119] Two measurements at different pH values are necessary for an exact correction, otherwise simplifications of the known equations have to be applied which do not hold over the whole pH range. The deviations from true values are particularly pronounced if the measurement is performed at pH values far different from the pK_a value of a given compound, where the correction equation tends to overshoot. An empirical equation developed in our laboratory using the tanh function may improve the situation (Table 2.3). For a direct correlation of HPLC-derived $\log k'_w$ values with $\log P_{oct}$ values, the measurement of some reference compounds with defined $\log P_{oct}$ values sometimes is recommended.

Micellar electrokinetic capillary chromatography (MEKC or MECC) is a further possibility for the determination of lipophilic properties. MEKC, firstly described by Terabe[120] is a special variant of capillary electrophoresis[121,122] (CE). Although the application of CE is generally limited to the measurement of ionized solutes, MEKC can be used for the separation of neutral solutes. The separation of neutral species is accomplished by the use of surfactants in the mobile buffer,[123] at concentrations above their critical micelle concentration. The surfactants and thus the formed micelles are charged and migrate in the capillary according to their charge. During the migration phase the solutes interact with the micelles through hydrophobic and electrostatic interactions. This method is predestined for the measurement of partition phenomena of compounds.[124] Since micelle systems are used in the separation, this might simulate the interaction with biological membranes in a better way than the common partition coefficients determined for 1-octanol/water. Recently two studies were published using MEKC[125] and microemulsion electrokinetic chromatography[126] (MEEKC) in the determination of lipophilic properties. A direct correlation with partition coefficients showed a good correlation between capacity factors from MEKC/MEEKC and log P_{oct} values. However only a few drug molecules were examined and these were mentioned to negatively influence the statistics of the correlation with log P_{oct} values. Moreover, only negatively charged micelle systems, which do not adequately mimic biological membranes, were used in these measurements. Ionized compounds show differences in their lipophilicity determined by MEKC/MEEKC in comparison to log P_{oct} values. Since most of the known drugs have ionizable groups, MEKC/MEEKC might be of great importance to further our understanding of drug membrane interactions. Further experimentation using MEKC with different more biomimetic micelle systems and more representative compound sets are required to assess the full potential of this new methodology.

LIPOPHILICITY CALCULATIONS

In principle two general methods for the calculation of partition coefficients have been reported. The first are fragment-based approaches using fragment constants derived from experimental lipophilicities. Hansch and Fujita[127,128] introduced a lipophilicity descriptor π (Equation 7), which was derived from the difference in log P_{oct} measurements of substituted and unsubstituted compounds. These π values are additive, so that the lipophilicity of a compound can be estimated using Equation 8.

$$\pi = \log P_{RX} - \log P_{RH} \tag{7}$$

$$\log P = \log P_{unsubstituted} + \sum_{1}^{n} \pi_{substituent_n} \tag{8}$$

The approach of Hansch has been extended and implemented in the computer program CLOGP, which is widely used in drug research and predicts $\log P_{oct}$ values reasonably well for compounds of limited conformational flexibility and structural complexity. Leo has recently reviewed this approach.[129] Another fragment-based approach, described by Rekker[130] (Equation 9), goes beyond the calculation of octanol/water partition coefficients. In this equation f_n is the hydrophobic fragment constant and a_n a numerical factor indicating the number of occurrences of a given fragment. Both methods have been extensively described and compared in different studies.[130-132]

Recently some new fragment-based calculation methods have been described by Klopman[133] and Convard.[134] Whether these methods offer major advantages to the established methods remains to be seen.

$$\log P = \sum_{1}^{n} a_n f_n + \text{correction terms} \tag{9}$$

For structurally or conformationally more complex compounds these fragment-based methods become unreliable. The problems arise from the fact, that the influence of conformation on lipophilicity is not handled adequately, that many important fragment values are still missing and that mutual interferences between fragments in a molecule are treated only for a small number of fragment interaction types.

Recently four approaches have been proposed using molecular surfaces[135-138] and so-called molecular lipophilicity potentials (MLP)[139] for the calculation of lipophilicities, giving reasonable correlations with experimental 1-octanol/water partition coefficients. In principle all these methods, as well as the approximate surface calculation (ASC)[140] developed in our laboratories, are using either total molecular surfaces, surface equivalents or grid points. Since these algorithms are based on the actual molecular geometry, lipophilicities are estimated as a function of conformation. These

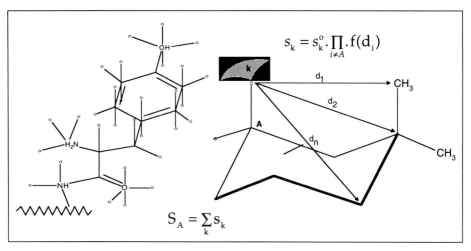

$$s_k = s_k^o \cdot \prod_{i \neq A} f(d_i)$$

$$S_A = \sum_k s_k$$

Fig. 2.5. The surface dot concept (ASC method/left). A small number of structure referenced surface points, called surface probes, are positioned around the atoms of a structure. The probe vectors are defined by hybridizations and ligand geometries of the atoms. Surface calculation using the ASC method (right). Surface equivalents S_k are assigned to the probe points, considering surface occlusions of overlapping neighboring atomic spheres using a simple distance function approach. The overall accessible surface S_A is defined by the sum of the surface equivalents S_k.

methods have the advantage to be scalable, are computationally very fast and do not depend on fragment values (Fig. 2.5). Unfortunately, 1-octanol/water is not a good system for the application of conformationally dependent partition coefficient calculations. Conformational estimates for a solute in the 1-octanol phase may be inadequate due to the high water content of the 1-octanol phase and its donor/acceptor properties, but for other organic solvents, like for example heptane, the calculation of conformation-dependent log P values represents an interesting approach, considering the hydrophobic collapse in the water phase and the hydrophilic collapse in the organic modifier (Fig. 2.6).

IONIZATION CONSTANTS (pK$_a$ values)

Looking through the different databases of known drugs, like the standard drug file (Derwent),[141] it is obvious that most of the compounds contain moieties which are charged under physiological conditions or can be charged in a pH range near the physiological pH. The ionization state of a compound strongly influences the different properties relevant to drug distribution and action. The introduction of a charged group can dramatically change the solubility. The lipophilicity of a compound and its transport through membranes depend on its ionization state. Therefore the ionization constant is an important property to be considered in the lead optimization process.

The ionization constant K_a (Equation 11) describes the equilibrium state for the deprotonation of a weak acid HA, as represented in Equation 10. The Henderson-Hasselbach Equation defines the relation between pH, pK_a and the ratio of protonated and deprotonated species (Equation 12). The ionization of a base can similarly be expressed by its pK_a value (Equation 13).

$$HA + H_2O \Leftrightarrow H_3O^+ + A^- \tag{10}$$

$$K_a = \frac{[H_3O^+][A^-]}{[HA]} \tag{11}$$

$$pH = pK_a + \log[BH^+]/[B] \tag{12}$$

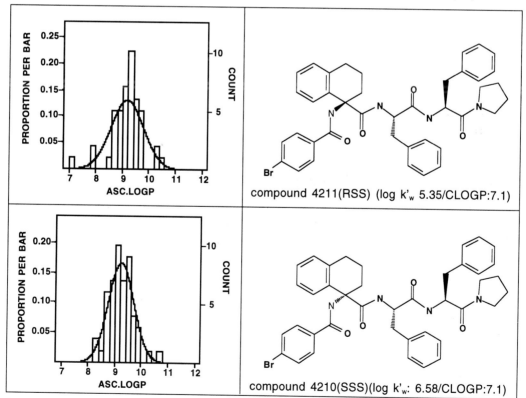

Fig. 2.6. Histogram of the ASC-LOGP distributions of a set of multiple conformers of two stereoisomers 4210 (bottom) and 4211 (top).

$$K_A = \frac{[B][H_3O^+]}{[BH^+]}$$
(13)

The literature of several methods for the measurement of pK_a values is described, including UV,[142] HPLC,[143,144] capillary zone electrophoresis (CZE),[145] solubility measurements[146,147] and potentiometric techniques.[148]

Although potentiometric techniques are known to have their limitations, they are the method of choice in most cases, since they are fast and give a complete overview of the ionization states of a compound over the whole pH range. The only major problem in the measurement of pK_a values of drugs, which is usually performed in water, is the often limited solubility of the compounds. This problem is further aggravated by the fact that potentiometric pK_a determinations are generally performed with the addition of ionic strength adjusters which may reduce drug solubility even further. For compounds with molecular weights up to 500 less than 0.5 mM solutions will be sufficient, the necessary amount is dependent on the expected pK_a values.[148] Often these concentrations cannot be reached in aqueous solution with a fixed ionic strength (e.g. aqueous 0.1 M KNO_3). Therefore the addition of organic solvents is often mandatory. However, the addition of organic solvent affects the pK_a value(s). In general, pK_a values for acids are shifted to higher values whereas pK_a values of basic groups are depressed. Avdeef and coworkers[96-98] could improve the methods described by Seiler[75] and Clarke[94] by introduction of special calibration methods and difference curve techniques. They could show that with minimum amounts of compounds a correct determination of pK_a values is still possible. Avdeef and coworkers could also demonstrate how a correct calibration with different organic solvent water ratios influences the result of the pK_a determination for a compound poorly soluble in water. Using these methods and newly developed equipment, the pK_a determination of poorly water-soluble compounds is straightforward, without the need for time consuming transfer of experimental data using external calculation programs.[149,150]

In addition, the potentiometric titration technique offers possibilities to determine other relevant molecular properties, such as log P_{oct} values of ionizable compounds, the stability constants of metal complexes, or the affinity of ionizable compounds to cyclodextrines or micellar systems.

ESTIMATION OF IONIZATION CONSTANTS

Calculation of pK_a values from molecular structure go back to the early work of Perrin, Dempsey and Serjeant[151] and Harris and Hayes.[152] Often a Hammett relationship is used for the calculation of pK_a and computer programs are available based on this methodology.[153] These programs seem to work well for simple structures, but for more complicated ones they usually fail. Rose and coworkers[154] compared the results of linear regression and neural network calculations of phenolic pK_a values using several property descriptors, the neural network being slightly better. Quantum mechanical methods[155,156] are used in the calculation of pK_a values. However the used pK_a data sets used were limited to a small number of simple compounds. The prediction of pK_a values has been reviewed by Perrin.[157]

As indicated above, the experimental measurement of pK_a values by potentiometric techniques is fast, but sometimes a complementary use of pK_a databases[158] and calculation methods may be helpful in assigning pK_a values to specific functional groups, especially if a compound exhibits several pK_a values, and also putting an experimental value into a broader structural perspective.

SOLUBILITY

DISSOLUTION RATES

When discussing solubilities of a compound one has to differentiate between the solubility itself and the dissolution rate as expressed by Equation 14.[159] The dissolution rate is a composite parameter and an important property for the bioavailability of a drug.

In a simple approximation, the dissolution rate can be expressed by the first order dissolution constant K and the maximum solubility of the compound, C_s, given by the concentration of a saturated solution.

$$\frac{dC}{dt} = K(C_s - C) \tag{14}$$

This simple equation has been extended including the surface area A of the dissolving particle (Equation 15), the diffusion coefficient for the compound D, the effective thickness of the diffusion layer h, and the volume of the dissolution medium V (Equation 16).[160,161] Other models for the description of dissolution rates have been described elsewhere.[162,163]

$$\frac{dC}{dt} = K_1 A (C_s - C_t) \tag{15}$$

$$\frac{dC}{dt} = \frac{K_2 DA}{Vh} (C_s - C_t) \tag{16}$$

Although the intrinsic solubility at defined conditions (e.g. pH/ionic strength) can not be modified, the dissolution rate can be enhanced in several ways:

- by increasing the effective surface area (micronization)
- by using surface active agents
- by a pH change (changing the chemical nature of the solute)
- by using solubility enhancers (e.g. cyclodextrins)

DESCRIPTION OF FACTORS INFLUENCING SOLUBILITY

Aqueous solubility is one of the key factors for the bioavailability of drugs. The aqueous solubility of a chemical is governed by three major factors:[177]

- intermolecular interactions in the crystal lattice
- the difference between the solute-water adhesive interaction and the sum of the solute-solute and water-water interactions
- the entropy of mixing (solute/solvent)

Accordingly, the solubility of a compound depends largely on its melting point and the molar enthalpy of fusion ΔH_f. Assuming an ideal solution, Equation 17 can be used to describe the solubility of a compound.

Table 2.4. Factors influencing results of solubility measurements

Solvent-based parameters	Solute parameters	Method-based parameters
solvent	crystal form/polymorphism	shaking time
pH of the solvent	counterions of solute	time between shaking and measurement (supersaturated solutions !)
ionic strength of the solvent	particle size	temperature
ionic strength adjuster itself		

$$\log\ X = -\frac{\Delta H_f}{2.303R}\left(\frac{T_0 - T}{T_0 T}\right) \tag{17}$$

Where X is the ideal solubility expressed as a mol fraction, T_0 is the melting point and T the absolute temperature of the solution. Galenical formulations of a drug often consist of a number of different components, resulting in less than ideal thermodynamic solutions. Therefore, Equation 17 cannot be used to calculate the solubility of a drug. In the case of a non-ideal solution the activity coefficient of the solute γ has to be considered (Equation 18). Thus, knowing the ideal solubility of a compound and its activity value, its solubility can be calculated. Nevertheless the calculated solubility often is not comparable with the measured values, since several important factors (Table 2.4) affect the experimental result.

$$\log X = -\frac{\Delta H_f}{2.303R}\left(\frac{T_0 - T}{T_0 T}\right) + \log\ \gamma \tag{18}$$

In order to calculate the activity coefficient γ, Scatchard[164] used the energy (w_2) required to release the solute molecule from the crystal surface, the energy of the cavity formation in the solvent (w_1), and the energy of the solvent solute interaction (w_{12}) according to Equation 19, where V is the molecular volume of the solute and Φ the volume fraction of the solute. In principle the solubility of a compound can thus be calculated from compound properties and parameters describing the cohesive effects between solvent and solute (surface tension, internal pressure, vaporization energy).

$$\log \gamma = (w_2 + w_1 - 2w_{12})\frac{V\Phi}{2.303RT} \tag{19}$$

The experimental determination of aqueous solubility seems to be a straightforward task. In practice however, there may be many pitfalls that should not be overlooked. The crystal form of the solute, its particle size, the ionic strength of the solvent are only a few parameters that may influence the result of a solubility measurement (Table 2.4). The influence of different salt forms have been extensively studied by several groups. Anderson and Conradi[165] examined the influence of counter ions on the solubility of anti-inflammatory acid flurbiprofen. Garren and Pyter[166] determined the influence of different salt concentrations on the solubility of renin inhibitors. 0.15 M NaCl salt solutions dramatically decrease the solubility of the examined inhibitors, however reverse effects are also described, for doxycycline derivatives.[167] An overview on criteria for an optimal salt selection for basic drugs is given by Gould.[168] In a new approach Serajuddin[169] describes the selection of salts considering different properties of a compound, including hygroscopicity, physical stability of crystal forms and aqueous solubility of different salts.

Most of the compounds under consideration have acidic/basic or zwitterionic properties. Therefore the pK_a of the solute and the pH of the solvent strongly influence the solubility. The solubility of acidic or basic compounds can therefore be used to determine the pK_a or vice versa. Albert[142] has described relationships between solubility and pK_a of acidic (Equation 20) or basic (Equation 21) solutes, where S_t is the observed solubility and S_i is the intrinsic solubility of the neutral compound. These equations allow to pre-assess the influences of pH on the solubility of a compound.

$$S_t = S_i \left(1 + \frac{K_a}{H^+} \right) = S_i \left(1 + 10^{(pH - pK_a)} \right) \tag{20}$$

$$S_t = S_i \left(1 + 10^{(pK_a - pH)} \right) \tag{21}$$

$$S_t = S_i \left(\frac{[H^+]^2 + K_1[H^+] + K_1 K_2}{K_1[H^+]} \right) \tag{22}$$

Using the simplified Equation 22, Ross and Riley[170] described the relation between pH and solubility for a set of zwitterionic diprotic quinoline compounds. With some exceptions the calculated solubilities showed a good correlation with the experimental values.

ESTIMATION OF SOLUBILITIES

Various attempts have been described in the literature to predict solubilities from the molecular structures. The different theoretical approaches for solubility predictions can be classified into methods based on:

- lipophilicity (log P_{oct}, CLOGP)
- lipophilicity and melting point
- molar surface and volume
- fragmental additivity schemes (group activity coefficients)

Simple equations have been derived showing a relationship between lipophilicity and aqueous solubility (S) or lipophilicity combined with melting point (mp) (Equations 23 and 24).

$$\log \frac{1}{S} = a \log P + b \tag{23}$$

$$\log S = -\log P - \Delta S_f \frac{(mp - 25)}{c} + d \tag{24}$$

These equations often hold only for series of congeneric compounds. Yalkowsky[171] and Valvani[172] obtained a semi-empirical relationship between aqueous solubility and octanol/water distribution coefficients and melting points for organic non-electrolytes (Equation 23). Using a larger compound set, including more than 40 drug molecules Tomlison and Hafkenscheid[173] demonstrated the advantage of using isocratic chromatographic HPLC retention parameters over partition coefficients. Good correlations were obtained with these equations within series of chemically similar compounds. A set of other prediction methods based on log P_{oct}, linear solubility energy relationships (LSER) and connectivity polarizability approaches have been summarized and tested by Speece et al.[174] Since these equations were derived and calibrated on small data sets, their predictive powers were found to be limited and extrapolations to larger data sets remain to be established. Most of these methods were only usable for compound subsets. In particular no drug molecules were included in the tests. The same is true for an extended study using connectivity indices.[175,176]

Based on the approximate relationship between solubility and log P_{oct} and the fact that log P_{oct} can be calculated from constitutional group contributions, Klopman et al[177] proposed a further group contribution approach using Equation 25, where S stands for the water solubility, the G_i represents the number of occurrences of groups i with associated solubility contribution factors a_i, a_0 being a solubility constant, introduced merely for improving statistics.

$$\log S = a_0 + \sum_{i=1}^{N} a_i G_i \tag{25}$$

Including a set of nine drug molecules a remarkable predictive power could be achieved. A similar approach has been proposed by Brüggemann and Altschuh.[178]

Jurs[179] used the ADAPT approach, to predict the solubilities of a set of nearly 300 compounds. Unfortunately no drug molecules were included. From the 157 descriptors used in his study, 45 were retained in the regression analysis and could be further condensed into 9 descriptors. However, a number of compounds had to be excluded from the data set. A good correlation between experimental and predicted solubilities could then be obtained. Similar results have been given by Suzuki[180] for another data set.

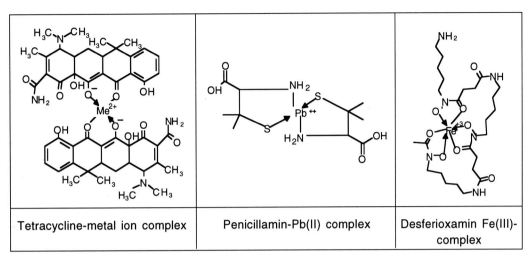

| Tetracycline-metal ion complex | Penicillamin-Pb(II) complex | Desferioxamin Fe(III)-complex |

Fig. 2.7. Examples of drug metal complexation.

In view of the many factors underlying solubility, it is not clear whether a reliable and generally applicable prediction method, comparable to the CLOGP calculation scheme, can be established. Therefore improved methodologies for efficient standardized measurements of solubilities are still needed. In this way extensive and representative solubility data sets would become available that could assist in the development of more generally applicable prediction schemes.

STABILITY CONSTANTS OF METAL COMPLEXES

The complexation of metal ions by biological relevant molecules plays an important role in many biochemical processes. Complexation of metals by drugs is known to affect their bioactivities (Fig. 2.7). The antibacterial activity of tetracyclines in chemotherapy is strongly influenced by complexation with metal ions like Mg^{2+}, Fe^{3+}, Al^{3+}, and Ca^{2+} ions.[181] Some gyrase inhibitors are known to bind Mg^{2+} weakly.[182] The metal complexation can be used to change physicochemical properties of a compound. Thus the solubility of a compound or the 1-octanol/water partition coefficient[183] can be influenced by metal complexation.

The thermodynamic stability of a metal-ion ligand complex $ML^{+(n-k)}$, formed by the interaction of a metal ion (M^{n+}) with a ligand (L^{k-}) as described by Equation 26, is given by the equilibrium or stability constant K according to Equation 27.

$$M^{n+} + L^{k-} \Leftrightarrow ML^{+(n-k)} \tag{26}$$

$$K = \frac{[ML^{+(n-k)}]}{[M^{n+}][L^{k-}]} \tag{27}$$

In aqueous solution the coordination sphere of a metal ion is usually fully occupied by water molecules so that ligand binding is a displacement reaction of one (or more) water molecules by one (or more) ligand molecules; however this is usually not explicitly formulated in equations like 26-30. A ligand is said to form a chelate, if two or more coordinated bonds can be formed to the metal ion generating a cyclic structure. The ligand is defined as unidentate if only one coordinate bond can be formed, and bidentate or multidentate if two or more coordinate bonds to the metal ion are possible.

Since metal ions usually have four or more coordination sites, they often bind more than one ligand. Metal-ligand complexation then generally involves several distinct complex species in thermodynamic equilibrium, each characterized by a specific complex stability constant. For example the binding of an amino acid like glycine to Cu^{2+} is described by the abbreviated two-step reaction scheme (Equations 28-29) with two stability constants as defined by Equations 30 and 31. In this reaction each ligand binding step is accompanied by the liberation of a proton. Therefore the equilibrium is strongly influenced by the pH of the solution and the pK_a value(s) of the ligand(s). The equilibrium constants described by Equations 30-31 are called stability constants, which do not consider the influence of the pK_a and pH, whereas the equilibrium constants which consider the pK_a values of the involved groups are called effective stability constants.

$$NH_3^+CHCOO^- + Cu^{2+} \Leftrightarrow Cu(NH_2CH_2COO)^+ + H^+ \tag{28}$$

$$Cu(NH_2CH_2COO)^+ + NH_3^+CHCOO^- \Leftrightarrow Cu(NH_2CH_2COO)_2 + H^+ \tag{29}$$

$$K_1 = \frac{[Cu(NH_2CH_2COO)^+]}{[Cu^{2+}][NH_2CH_2COO^-]} \qquad (30)$$

$$K_2 = \frac{[Cu(NH_2CH_2COO)_2]}{[Cu(NH_2CH_2COO)^+][NH_2CH_2COO^-]} \qquad (31)$$

The stepwise stability constants, are often summarized and expressed by cumulative or overall stability constants, beta-values, being the products of the stepwise stability constants, i.e., $\beta_1 = K_1$, $\beta_2 = K_1 \ast K_2$. Taking the above example $\log \beta_1 = \log K_1 = 8.28$ and $\log \beta_2 = \log K_1 + \log K_2 = 15.16$.

For complexation reactions in ionic strength-adjusted water, stability constants are not adequate to describe the actual situation. In most cases, competition reactions of the protons in solution have to be considered. This leads to the so-called terms of the effective or conditional stability constants described by Equations 32 and 33, where the pK_a value(s) of the ligand(s) are considered.

$$\log K_{ML}^{eff} = \log K_{ML} - \log a_L \qquad (32)$$

Table 2.5. Analytical methods for the determination of formation constants of metal complexes

Potentiometry

Nuclear magnetic resonance spectroscopy

Polarography

Ion exchange measurements

Colorimetry

Ionic conductivity

Distribution between two phases

Solubility measurements

Partial pressure measurements (for volatile ligands)

UV-spectroscopy

(Reproduced with permission from: Martell AE, Motekaitis RJ. In: Determination and Use of Stability constants. 2nd ed., New York: VCH, ©1992.)

where

$$a_L = 1 + \sum_{i=i}^{N} \beta_i^H [H^+]^i \tag{33}$$

Knowing the different ionization constants β_i^H of a compound, the effective stability constants can be easily calculated using Equations 32 and 33.

Generally any method which provides the concentration of at least one equilibrium species together with the known solution conditions can be used to determine equilibrium constants. Table 2.5[184] gives an overview of the different methods that can be used for the determination of stability constants. The measurement of stability constants of metal complexes by the potentiometric titration method is particularly useful and has been described by several groups.[184-186]

Using the increasing number of known metal complex equilibrium constants,[187] several group-contribution methods for the prediction of equilibrium constants, have been derived.[184] The most successful method appears to be the one reported by Harris,[184] which is based on an additivity scheme for functional group values with correction terms for chelate formation.

CONCLUSION AND OUTLOOK

Pharmaceutical industry undergoes rapid changes. The increased hurdles for innovation call for a significant reduction in cost and time for the drug discovery and development process. One important issue is the early incorporation of pharmacologically relevant physicochemical and biophysical compound properties into the process of lead optimization. This calls for further refinements of existing methodologies for the experimental measurement of relevant properties. It also calls for continued efforts to identify new parameters that closely correlate with relevant aspects of in vivo bioavailability. In parallel with experimental methods, computational schemes have to be refined for adequate estimates of relevant compound properties so that extensive compound sets can be assessed reliably even if generated only by computer.

With the advent of combinatorial chemistry and the possibility to produce large collections of individual compound sets, methodologies for adequately estimating pharmacologically relevant compound properties will be very important in the planning of libraries with designed molecular diversity, but new analytical techniques have to be devised also to allow the experimental determination of physicochemical or biophysical parameters in parallel for large numbers of compounds available only in small quantities. These are interesting areas of both technological, methodological and conceptual innovations. They will undoubtedly happen in the near future and will have substantial impact on the overall drug discovery and development process.

REFERENCES

1. Seydel JK, Schaper KJ. Chemische Struktur und Biologische Aktivität von Wirkstoffen, Weihnheim: Verlag Chemie, 1979.
2. Martin EJ, Blaney JM, Siani MA et al. Measuring diversity: experimental design of combinatorial libraries for drug discovery. J Med Chem 1995; 38:1431-1436.
3. Martin YC. 3D database searching in drug design. J Med Chem 1992; 35:2145-2154.
4. Kuntz ID. Structure-based strategies for drug design and discovery. Science 1992; 257:1078-1082.
5. Pearlman RS. 3D molecular structures: generation and use in 3D searching. In: Kubinyi H, ed. 3D QSAR in Drug Design. Leiden: Escom, 1993:41-80.
6. Van Drie JH, Weininger D, Martin YC. ALADDIN: An integrated tool for computer-assisted molecular design and pharmacophore recognition from geometric, steric and substructure searching of three dimensional molecular structures. J Comput-Aided Mol Des 1989; 3:255-251.
7. Greene J, Kahn S, Savoj H et al. Chemical function queries for 3D database searching. J Chem Inf Comput Sci 1994; 34:1297-1308.
8. Schaper KJ Absorption of ionizable drugs: nonlinear dependence on log P pKa and pH-quantitative relationships. Quant Struct-Act Relat 1982; 1:13-27.
9. Kubinyi H. History and development of QSAR. In: Wolf E ed. Medicinal Chemistry and Drug Discovery. Volume 1: Principles and Practice. 5th ed. New York: Willey & Sons, 1995:498-569.
10. Kubinyi H. Parameters. In: Mannhold R, Krogsgaard L, Timmerman H, eds. QSAR: Hansch Analysis and Related Approaches. Weinheim: VCH, 1993:21-54.

11. Jurs PC, Dixon SL, Leanne ME. Representations of molecules. In: van de Waterbeemd H, ed. Methods and Principles in Medicinal Chemistry: Volume 2. Chemometric Methods in Molecular Design. Weinheim: VCH, 1995:15-38.

12. Hansch C, Leo A. Exploring QSAR. Washinghton DC: ACS Professional Reference Book, 1995.

13. Bowden K. Electronic effects in drugs. In: Hansch C, Sammes G, Taylor JB eds. Comprehensive Medicinal Chemistry: Volume 4: Quantitative Drug Design. Oxford: Pergamon Press, 1990:205-239.

14. Taylor PJ. Hydrophobic properties of drugs. In: Hansch C, Sammes G, Taylor JB eds. Comprehensive Medicinal Chemistry: Volume 4: Quantitative Drug Design. Oxford: Pergamon Press, 1990: 241-294.

15. Silipo C, Vittoria A. Three-dimensional structure of drugs. In: Hansch C, Sammes G, Taylor JB eds. Compensive Medicinal Chemistry: Volume 4: Quantitative Drug Design. Oxford: Pergamon Press, 1990:153-204.

16. Hansch C, Leo A, Hoekman D. Exploring QSAR. Hydrophobic, Electronic, and Steric constants. Washinghton DC: ACS Professional Reference Book, 1995.

17. van de Waterbeemd H, Testa B. The parametrization of lipophilicity and other structural properties in drug research. Adv Drug Res 1987; 16:85-225.

18. TSAR V2.3, Oxford Molecular Ltd., The Magdalen Centre, Oxford Science Park, Oxford OX4 4GA, UK.

19. Franke R, Gruska A. Multivariate data analysis of chemical and biological data. In: van de Waterbeemd H, ed. Methods and Principles in Medicinal Chemistry. Volume 2. Chemometric Methods in Molecular Design. Weinheim: VCH, 1995:111-163.

20. Wold S. PLS for multivariate linear modeling. In: van de Waterbeemd H, ed. Methods and Principles in Medicinal Chemistry. Volume 2: Chemometric Methods in Molecular Design. Weinheim: VCH, 1995:195-218.

21. Dunn WJ, Wold S. SIMCA pattern recognition and classification. In: van de Waterbeemd H, ed. Methods and Principles in Medicinal Chemistry. Volume 2: Chemometric Methods in Molecular Design. Weinheim: VCH, 1995:179-193.

22. Sjöström M, Eriksson L. Applications of statistical experimental design and PLS modeling in QSAR. In: van de Waterbeemd H, ed. Methods and Principles in Medicinal Chemistry. Volume 2: Chemometric Methods in Molecular Design. Weinheim: VCH, 1995:111-163.

23. Shepard RN, Romney AK, Nerlove S. Multidimensional Scaling: Theory and Application in the Behavioral Sciences. New York, Academic Press: 1972.

24. Schiffmann SS, Reynolds ML, Young FW. Introduction to Multi-dimensional Scaling: Theory, Methods, and Applications. New York, Academic Press 1981.

25. van de Waterbeemd H, Constantino G, Clementi et al. Disjoint principle properties of organic substituents. In: van de Waterbeemd H, ed. Chemometric Methods in Molecular Design. Weinheim; VCH, 1995:103-112.

26. Kubinyi H. Variable selection in QSAR studies. I. An evolutionary algorithm. Quant Struct-Act Relat 1994; 13:285-294.

27. Kubinyi H. Variable selection in QSAR studies. II. A highly efficient combination of systematic search and evolution. Quant Struct-Act Relat 1994; 13:393-401.

28. Kier LB, Hall LH. Molecular Connectivity in Chemistry and Drug Research. London, Academic Press, 1976.

29. Kier LB, Hall LH. Molecular Connectivity in Structure-Activity Analysis. London, John Wiley, 1986.

30. Kier LB. Atom-level descriptors for QSAR analyzes. In: van de Waterbeemd H, ed. Chemometric Methods in Molecular Design. Weinheim: VCH, 1995:39-47.

31. Hall LH, Mohney BK, Kier LB. Comparison of electrotopological state index with parameters: inhibition of MAO by hydrazides. Quant Struct Act Relat 1993; 12:44-48.

32. Llorente B, Rivero N, Carrasco R et al. A QSAR study of quinolones based on electrotopological state index from atoms. Quant Struct Act Relat 1994; 13:419-422.

33. Kubinyi H. QSAR: Hansch analysis and related approaches. In: Mannhold R, Krogsgaard-Larsen P, Timmermann H, eds. Methods and Principles in Medicinal Chemistry. Volume 1: Weinheim: VCH, 1993.

34. El Tayar N, Tsai RS, Testa B et al. Partitioning of solutes in different solvent systems: the contribution of hydrogen-bonding capacity and polarity. J Pharm Sci 1991; 80:590-598.

35. Raevsky O, Grigor'ev V, Mednikova E. QSAR H-bonding descriptions. In: Wermuth CG, ed. Trends in QSAR and Molecular Modelling 92. Leiden, Escom: 1993:116-119.

36. Abraham MH, Duce PP, Prior DV et al. Hydrogen bonding. Part 9. Solute proton donor and proton acceptor scales for use in drug design. J Chem Soc Perkin Trans II 1989:1355-1375.

37. Abraham MH, Chadha HS, Whiting GS et al. Hydrogen bonding. 32. An analysis of water-octanol and water-alkane partitioning and Δlog P parameter of Seiler. J Pharm Sci 1994; 83:1994.

38. Hansch C, Leo A. Substituent Constants for Correlation Analysis in Chemistry and Biology, New York: Wiley, 1979.

39. Van de Waterbeemd H, Kansy M. Brain penetration and H-bonding capacity. In: Wermuth CG, ed. Trends in QSAR and Molecular Modelling 92. Leiden: Escom, 1993:550-551.

40. Lien EJ, Guo ZR, Li RL. Use of dipole moments as a parameter in drug-receptor interactions and quantitative strcture-activity relationship studies. J Pharm Sci 1982; 71:641-655.

41. Lien EJ, Guo ZR, Li RL et al. Examination of the interrelationship between aliphatic group dipole moment and polar substituent constants. J Pharm Sci 1984; 73:553-558.

42. Lien EJ, Liao RCH, Shinouda HG. Quantitative structure-activity relationships and dipole moments of anticonvulsants and CNS depressants. J Pharm Sci 1979; 68:463-465.

43. Oprea TI, Kurunczi L, Moret EE. Role of the dipole moment during ligand receptor interaction. A hypothetic static model. In: Wermuth CG, ed. Trends in QSAR and Molecular Modelling 92. Leiden: Escom Science Publishers, 1993:398-399.

44. Pearlmann RS, Molecular surface areas and volumes and their use in structure-activity relationships. In: Yalkowsky SH, Sikula AA, Valvani SC, eds. Physical Chemical Properties of Drugs. New York: Marcel Dekker, 1980:321-345.

45. Lee B, Richards FM. The interpretation of protein structures: estimation of static accessibility. J Mol Bio 1971; 55:379-400.

46. Silla E, Tunon I, Pascual-Ahuir JL. GEPOL: an improved description of molecular surfaces. II. Computing the molecular area and volume. J Comput Chem 1991; 12:1077-1088.

47. Pearlmann RS. Molecular surface areas and volumes: their calculations and use in predicting solubilities and free energies of dissolution. In: Dunn WJ, Block JH, Pearlmann RS, eds. Partition Coefficient Determination and Estimation. New York: Pergamon Press, 1986:3-10.

48. Koehler MG, Grigorias S, Dunn III WJ. The relationship between chemical structure and the logarithm of the partition coefficient. Quant Struct-Act Relat 1988; 7:150-159.

49. Dearden JC. Molecular structure and drug transport. In: Hansch C, Sammes G, Taylor JB. eds. Comprehensive Medicinal Chemistry: Volume 4: Quantitative Drug Design. Oxford: Pergamon Press, 1990:375-411.

50. Bunge AL, Cleek LR. A new method for estimating dermal absorption from chemical exposure: 2. Effect of molecular weight and octanol-water partitioning. Pharm Res 1995; 12:88-95.

51. CATALYST V2.3. Molecular Simulations. 16 New England Executive Park, Burlington, Massachusetts, USA 01803.

52. Thomson C. The use of quantum chemistry in the study of biological problems. Chem Des Automation News 1994; 9(5):1-30.

53. Dewar MJS, Thiel W. Ground states of molecules. 38. The MNDO method. Approximations and parameters. J Am Chem Soc 1977; 99:4899-4907.

54. Dewar MJS, Zoebisch EG, Healy et al. AM1: a new general purpose quantum mechanical molecular model. J Am Chem Soc 1985; 107:3902-3909.

55. Smith RP, Ree T, Magee JL et al. The inductive effect and chemical reactivity. I. General theory of the inductive effect and application to electic dipole moments of haloalkanes. J Am Chem Soc 1951; 73:2263-2267.

56. Debnath AK, Lopez de Compadre RL, Debnath G et al. Structure-activity relationships of mutagenic aromatic and heteroaromatic nitro compounds. Correlation with molecular orbital energies and hydrophobicity. J Med Chem 1991; 34:786-797.

57. Gasteiger J, Marsili M. Iterative partial equalization of orbital electronegativity- a rapid access to atomic charges. Tetrahedron 1980; 36:3219-3228.

58. Gasteiger J, Hutchings MG, Christoph B et al. A new treatment of chemical reactivity: development of EROS, an expert system for reaction prediction and synthesis design. Topics Curr Chem 1987; 137:19-73.

59. Dixon SL, Jurs PC. Atomic charge for quantitative structure-propery relationships. J Comput Chem 1992; 4:492-504.

60. Kubinyi H. Free Wilson analysis. Theory, applications and its relationship to Hansch analysis. Quant Struct-Act Relat 1988; 7:121-133.

61. Dunn WJ, Wold S. Statistical analysis of the partition coefficients. Acta Chem Scand 1978, B32:536-542.

62. Franke R, Kühne R, Dove S. Dependence of hydrophobicity on solvent and structure. In: Dearden JC, ed. Quantitative Approaches to Drug Design. Amsterdam: Elsevier, 1983:15-32.

63. Alcorn CJ, Simpson RJ, Leahy D et al. In vitro studies of intestinal drug absorption. Determination of partition and distribution coefficients with brush border membrane vesicles. Biochem Pharmacol 1991; 42:2259-2264.

64. Alcorn CJ, Simpson RJ, Leahy D et al. Partition and distribution coefficients of solutes and drugs in brush border membrane vesicles. Biochem Pharmacol 1993:1775-1782.

65. Thomas PG, Seelig J. Binding of the calcium antagonist flunarizine to phosphatidylcholine bilayers: charge effects and thermodynamics. Biochem J 1993; 291:397-402.

66. Herbette LG, Chester DW, Rhodes DG. Structural analysis of drug molecules in biological membranes. Biophys J 1986; 49:91-94.

67. Mason RP, Rhodes DG, Herbette LG. Reevaluating equilibrium and kinetic binding parameters from lipophilic drugs based on a structural model for drug interaction with biological membranes. J Med Chem 1991; 34:869-877.

68. Young HS, Mason RP, Herbette LG. Molecular basis for drug-drug interactions in cardiac sarcolemmal membranes. Biophys J 1990; 57:523a.

69. Herbette LG, Rhodes DG, Mason RP. New approaches to drug design and delivery based on drug-membrane interactions. Drug Des Delivery 1991; 7:75-118.

70. Seydel JK, Albores Velasco M, Coats EA et al. The importance of drug-membrane interaction in drug research and development. Quant Struct-Act Relat 1992; 11:205-210.

71. Murthy KS, Zografi G. Oil-water partitioning of chlorpromazine and other phenothiazine derivatives using dodecane and n-octanol. J Pharm Sci 1970; 9:1281-1285.

72. Leahy DE, Taylor PJ, Wait AR. Model solvent systems for QSAR Part I. Propylene glycol dipelargonate (PGDP). A new standard solvent for use in partition coefficient determination. Quant Struct-Act Relat 1989; 8:17-31.

73. Collander R. The partition of organic compounds between higher alcohols and water. Acta Chem Scand 1951; 5:774-780.

74. Seiler P. Interconversions of lipophilicities from hydrocarbon/water systems into octanol/water systems. Eur J Med Chem 1974; 9; 473-479.

75. Seiler P. The simultaneous determination of partition coefficients and acidity constants of a substance. Eur J Med Chem 1974; 9:663-666.

76. Young RC, Mitchell RC, Brown TH et al. Development of a new physicochemical model for brain penetration and its application to the design of centrally acting H_2 receptor histamine antagonists. J Med Chem 1988; 31:656-671.

77. van de Waterbeemd H, Kansy M. Hydrogen-bonding capacity and brain penetration. Chimia 1992:299-303.

78. Testa B, Seiler P. Steric and lipophilic components of hydrophobic fragmental constants. Arzneim Forsch (Drug Res) 1981; 31:1053-1058.

79. El Tayar N, Testa B, Carrupt PA. Polar intermolecular interactions encoded in partition coefficients: an indirect estimation of hydrogen-bond parameters of polyfunctional solutes. J Phys Chem 1992; 96:1455-1459.

80. Paterson DA, Conradi RA, Hilgers AR et al. A non-aqueous partitioning system for predicting the oral absorption potential of peptides. Quant Struct-Act Relat 1994; 13:4-10.

81. Hovgaard L, Brøndstedt H, Buur A et al. Drug delivery studies in caco-2 monolayers. Synthesis, hydrolysis, and transport of O-cyclopropane carboxylic acid ester prodrugs of various β-blocking agents. Pharm Res 1995; 12:387-392.

82. Dearden JC, Bresnen G. The measurement of partition coefficients. Quant Struct-Act Relat 1988; 7:133-144.

83. El Tayar N, Marston A, Bechalany A et al. Use of centrifugal partition chromatography for assessing partition coefficients in various solvent systems. J Chromatogr 1989; 469:91-99.

84. El Tayar N, Tsai RS, Vallat P, Altomare C, Testa B. Measurement of partition coefficients by various centrifugal partition chromatographic techniques. J Chromatogr 1991; 665:181-194.

85. Berthod A, Menges RA, Amstrong DW. Direct octanol water partition coefficient determination using co-current chromatography. J Liq Chromatogr 1992; 15:2769-2785.

86. Conway WD. Counter-current chromatography. J Chromatogr 1991; 538:27-35.

87. Tsai R-S, El Tayar N, Testa B. Toridal coil centrifugal partition chromatography, a method for measuring partition coefficients. J Chromatogr 1991; 538:119-123.

88. Ito Y. Recent advances in counter-current chromatography. J Chromatogr 1991:3-25.

89. Foucault AP. Countercurrent chromatography. Anal Chem 1991; 63:569-579.

90. Barnett SP, Hill AP, Livingstone DJ et al. A new method for calculation of partition coefficients from experimental data for both mixtures and pure compounds. Quant Struct-Act Relat 1992; 11:505-509.

91. Hersey A, Hill AP, Hyde RM, Livingstone J. Principles of method selection in partition studies. Quant Struct-Act Relat 1989; 8:288-296.

92. Avdeef A, Comer EA. Measurement of pK_a and log P of water-insoluble substances by potentiometric titration. In: Wermuth CG, ed. Trends in QSAR and Molecular Modelling 92. Leiden: Escom Science Publishers, 1993:386-387.

93. Brandstöm A. A rapid method for the determination of distribution coefficient of bases for biological purposes. Acta Chem Scand 1963; 17:1218-1224.

94. Clarke FH. Ionization constants by curve fitting: Application to the determination of partition coefficients. J Pharm Sci 1984; 226-230.

95. Clarke FH, Cahoon NM. Ionization constants by curve fitting: Determination of partition and distribution coefficients of acids and bases and their ions. J Pharm Sci 1987; 8:611-620.

96. Avdeef A. pH-metric log P. Part 1. Difference plots for determining ion-pair octanol water partition coefficients of multiprotic substances. Quant Struct-Act Relat 1992; 11:510-517.

97. Avdeef A. pH-metric log P. II: Refinement of partition coefficients and ionization constants of multiprotic substances. J Pharm Sci 1993; 82:183-190.

98. Avdeef A, Comer JEA, Thomson SJ. pH-metric log P. 3. Glass electrode calibration in methanol-water, applied to pK_a determinations of water-insoluble substances. Anal Chem 1993; 65:42-49.

99. Slater B, McCormack A, Avdeef A et al. pH-metric log P. 4. Comparison of partition coefficients determined by HPLC and potentiometric methods to literature values. J Pharm Sci 1994; 9: 1280-1283.

100. Dross K, Sonntag C, Mannhold R. Determination of hydrophobicity parameter R_{MW} by reversed phase thin-layer chromatography. J Chromatogr 1994; 673, 113-124.

101. Hafkenscheid TL, Tomlinson E. Estimation of physicochemical properties of organic solutes using HPLC retention parameters. Adv Chromatogr 1986; 25:1-62.

102. Gaspari F, Bonatti M. Correlation between n-octanol/water partition coefficient and liquid chromatographic retention for caffeine and ist metabolites, and some structure-pharmacokinetic considerations. J Pharm Pharmacol 1987; 39:252-260.

103. Kaliszan R. High performance liquid chromatographic methods and procedures of hydrophobicity determinations. Quant Struct-Act Relat 1990; 9:83-87.

104. Zou H, Zhang Y, Hong M, Lu P. Measurement of partition coefficients by reversed-phase ion-pair liquid chromatography. J Chromatogr 1992; 625:169-175.

105. Biagi GL, Barbaro AM, Sapone A et al. Determination of lipophilicity by means of reversed-phase thin-layer chromatography. II Influence of the organic modifier on the slope of the thin-layer chromatographic equation. J Chromatogr 1994; 669:246-253.

106. Dorsey JG, Khaledi MG. Hydrophobicity estimations by reversed-phase chromatography. Implications for biological partitioning processes. J Chromatogr A 1993; 656:485-499.

107. Lambert WJ. Modelling oil-water partitioning and membrane permeation using reversed-phase chromatography. J Chromatogr A 1993; 656:469-484.

108. Schoenmakers PJ, Billiet HAH, Tijssen R et al. Gradient selection in reversed-phase liquid chromatography. J Chromatogr 1978; 149:519-537.

109. Schoenmakers PJ, Billiet HAH, Tijssen R et al. Influence of organic modifiers on the retention behaviour in reversed-phase liquid

chromatography and ist consequences for gradient elution. J Chromatogr 1979; 185:179-195.

110. El Tayar N, van de Waterbeemd H, Testa B. Lipophilicity measurements of protonated basic compounds by reversed-phase high performance liquid chromatography. I. Relationship between capacity factors and the methanol concentration in methanol-water eluents. J Chromatogr 1985; 320:293-304.

111. Unger SH, Cook JR, Hollenberg JS. Simple procedure for determining octanol-aqueous partition, distribution, and ionization coefficients by reversed-phase high-pressure liquid chromatography. J Pharm Sci 1978; 67:1364-1366.

112. Bechalany A, Tsantili-Kakoulidou A, El Tayar N et al. Measurement of lipophilicity indices by reversed-phase high performance liquid chromatography: comparison of two stationary phases and various eluents. J Chromatogr 1991; 541:221-229.

113. Vallat P, Fan W, El Tayar N et al. Solvatochromic analysis of the retention mecganism of two novel stationary phases used for measuring lipophilicity by RP-HPLC. J Liq Chromatogr 1992; 15:2133-2151.

114. Pidgeon C, Marcus C, Alvarez F. Immobilized artificial membrane chromatography: surface chemistry and applications. In: Kelly JW, Baldwin TO, eds. Applications of Enzyme Biotechnology, New York: Plenum Press, 1991:201-219.

115. Pidgeon C, Venkataram UV. Immobilized artificial membrane chromatography: supports composed of membrane lipids. Analyt Biochem 1989; 176:36-47.

116. Pidgeon C, Ong S, Liu H, Qiu X et al. IAM Chromatography: an in vitro screen for predicting drug membrane permeability. J Med Chem 1995; 38:590-594.

117. Ong S, Cai SJ, Bernal C et al. Phospholipid immobilization on solid surfaces. Anal Chem 1994; 66:782-792.

118. Kaliszan R, Nasal A, Bucinski A. Chromatographic hydrophobicity parameter determined on an immobilized artifical membrane column: relationship to standard measures of hydrophobicity and bioactivity. Eur J Med Chem 1994; 29(2):163-170.

119. Horvath C, Melander W, Molnar I. Liquid chromatography of ionogenic substances with nonpolar stationary phases. Anal Chem 1977; 49:142-154.

120. Terabe S. Electrokinetic chromatography: an interface between electrophoresis and chromatography. Trends Anal Chem 1989; 8:129-134.

121. Li SFY. Capillary Electrophoresis: Principles, Practice and Applications, 1st ed. Elsevier: Amsterdam, 1992.

122. Monning CA, Kennedy RT, Capillary electrophoresis. Anal Chem 1994; 280R-314R.

123. Swedberg SA. Use of non-ionic and zwitterionic surfactants to enhance selectivity in high performance capillary electrophoresis. An apparent micellar electrokinetic capillary chromatography mechanism. J Chromatogr 1990; 503:449-452.

124. Weinberger R, Lurie IS. Micellar electrokinetic capilary chromatography of illicit drug substances. Anal Chem 1991; 63:823-827.

125. Bradford JH, Dorsey JG. n-Octanol-water partition coefficient estimation by micellar electrokinetic capillary chromatography. Anal Chem 1995; 67:744-749.

126. Ishihama Y, Oda Y, Uchikawa K et al. Evaluation of solute hydrophobicity by microemulsion electrokinetic chromatography. Anal Chem 1995; 67:1588-1595.

127. Hansch C, Maloney PM, Fujita T et al. Correlation of biological activity of phenoxyacatic acids with Hammett substituent constants and partition coefficients. Nature 1962; 194:178-180.

128. Hansch C, Fujita T. ρ–σ–π Analysis. A method for the correlation of biological activity and chemical structure. J Am Chem Soc 1964; 86:1616-1626.

129. Leo AJ. Calculating log P_{oct} from structures. Chem Reviews 1993; 4:1283-1305.

130. Mannhold R, Dross KP, Rekker RF. Drug Lipophilicity in QSAR practice: I. A comparison of experimental with calculative approaches. Quant Struct-Act Relat 1990; 9:21-28.

131. Mayer JM, van de Waterbeemd H, Testa B. A comparison between the hydrophobic fragmental method of Rekker and Leo. Eur J Med Chem 1982; 17:17-25.

132. Mannhold R, Rekker RF, ter Laak AM. On the reliability of calculated log P-values: Rekker-, Hansch/Leo- and Suzuki-approach. In: Wermuth CG, ed. Trends in QSAR and molecular modelling 92. Leiden: Escom Science Publishers, 1993:379-380.

133. Klopman G, Li J-Y, Wang S, Dimayuga M. Computer automated log P calculations on an extended group contribution approach. J Chem Inf Comput Sci 1994; 34:752-781.

134. Convard T, Dubost J-P, Solleu H et al. Smilog P: a program for a fast evaluation of theoretical log P from the smiles code of a molecule. Quant Struct-Act Relat 1994; 13:34-37.

135. Pixner P, Heiden W, Merx H et al. Empirical method for the quantification and localization of molecular hydrophobicity. J Chem Inf Comput Sci 1994; 34:1309-1319.

136. van de Waterbeemd H, Karajiannis H, Kansy M et al. Conformation-lipophilicity relationships of peptides and peptide mimetics. In: Sanz F, ed. Trends in QSAR and Molecular Modeling 94, Barcelona: Prous, in press.

137. Richards NGJ, Williams PB. Conformation-dependent partition coefficient calculations. Chem Des Automation News 1994; 9:1-26.

138. Carrupt P. Conformation-dependent log P calculation from the molecular lipophilicity potential. In: Pliska V, Testa B, van de Waterbeemd H eds. Lipophilicity in Drug Action and Toxicology, Weinheim: VCH, in press.

139. Gaillard P, Carrupt PA, Testa B et al. Molecular lipophilicity potential, a tool in 3D QSAR. Method and applications. J Comput-Aided Mol Design 1994; 8:83-96.

140. Ulmschneider M. Analytical model for the calculation of van der Waals and solvent accessible surface areas. Contribution to the calculation of free enthalpies of hydration and octanol/water partition coeffiecients. Thesis 1993, Université de Haute-Alsace, Mulhouse, France.

141. Standard Drug File, Derwent Publications, Rochdale House, 128 Theobald Road, London, WC1X 8RP, UK.

142. Albert A, Serjeant EP. The Determination of Ionization Constants. A Laboratory Manual. 3rd ed. London: Chapman and Hall, 1984.

143. Miyake K, Okumura K, Terada H. Determination of acid dissociation constants by high-performance liquid chromatography. Chem Pharm Bull 1985; 33:769-777.

144. Hafkenscheid TL. Influences of the mobile phase methanol content on the relationship between reversed-phase liquid chromatographic retention of aromatic compounds. J Chromatogr Sci 1986; 24:307-316.

145. Gluck SJ, Cleve JA. Investigation of experimental approaches to the determination of pK_a values by capillary electrophoresis. J Chromatogr 1994; 680:49-56.

146. Zimmermann I. Determination of overlapping pK_a values from solubility data. Int J Pharm 1986; 31:69-74.

147. Peck CC, Benet LZ. Determining macrodissociation constants of polyprotic amphoteric compounds from solubility measurements. Int J Pharm 1978; 67:1,12-16.

148. Comer JEA, Avdeef A, Box KJ. Limits for successful measurement of pK_a and log P by pH-metric titration. Am Lab 1995:36C-37H.

149. Meloun M, Havel J, Högefeldt E. Computation of Solution Equilibria. A Guide to Methods in Potentiometric Extraction, and Spectrophotometry. New York: John Wiley, 1988.

150. Havel J, Meloun M. General computer programs for the determination of formation constants from various types of data. In: Legget DJ, ed. Computational Methods for the Determination of Formation Constants. New York: Plenum Press, 1985:221-289.

151. Perrin D, Dempsey B, Serjeant E. pKa Prediction for Organic Acids and Bases.London: Chapman & Hall, 1981.

152. Harris J, Hayes M. Handbook of Chemical Property Estimations Methods. New York: McGraw-Hill, 1981.

153. Csizmadia F, Szegezdi J, Darvas F. Expert system for predicting pK$_a$. In: Wermuth CG, ed. Trends in QSAR and Molecular Modelling 92. Leiden: Escom Science Publishers, 1993:499-501.

154. Rose VS, Hill AP, Hyde RM, Hersey A. pK$_a$ prediction in multiply-substituted phenols: A comparison of multiple linear regression and back-propagation. In: Wermuth CG, ed. Trends in QSAR and Molecular Modelling 92. Leiden: Escom Science Publishers, 1993:499-501.

155. Gruber C, Buss V. Quantum-mechanically calculated properties for the development of quantitative structure-activity relationships (QSAR's). pKa-values of phenols and aromatic and aliphatic carboxylic acids. Chemosphere 1989; 19:1595-1609.

156. Dixon SL, Jurs PC. Estimation of pKa for organic oxyacids using calculated atomic charges. J Comp Chem 1993; 14:1460-1467.

157. Perrin DD. The prediction of pK$_a$-values. In: Yalkowsky SH, Sinkula AA, Valvani SC, eds. Physical Properties of Drugs. New York: Marcel Dekker, 1980:2-48.

158. MEDCHEM95B, Daylight Chemical Information Systems, 18500 von Karman Avenue, Irvine, CA 92715, USA.

159. Noyes AA, Whitney WR. The rate of solution of solid substances in their own solutions. J Am Chem Soc 1897; 19:930-934.

160. Abdou HM. Dissolution, Bioavailability, and Bioequivalence. Easton: Mack Publishing Company, 1989.

161. Grant DJW, Higuchi T. Solubility behavior of organic compounds. In: Saunders WH, Weissberger A, eds. Techniques of Chemistry. Volume XXI. New York. Wiley & Sons, 1990.

162. Danckwerts PV. Significance of liquid-film coefficients in gas absorption. Ind Eng Chem 1951; 43:1460-1467.

163. Higuchi WI. Diffusional models useful in biopharmaceutics. Drug release rate processes. J Pharm Sci 1967; 56:315-324.

164. Scatchard G. Equilibria in non-electrolyte solutions in relation to the vapor pressures and densities of the components. Chem Rev 1931; 8:321-333.

165. Anderson BD, Conradi RA. Predictive relationships in the water solubility of salts of a nonsteroidal anti-inflammatory drug. J Pharm Sci 1985; 74:815-820.

166. Garren KW, Pyter RA. Aqueous solubility properties of a dibasic peptide-like compound. Int J Pharm 1990; 63:167-172.

167. Bogardus JB, Blackwood RK. Solubility of doxycycline in aqueous solution. Pharm Sci 1979; 86:188-194.

168. Gould PL. Salt selection for basic drugs. Int J Pharm 1986; 33: 201-217.

169. Morris KR, Fakes MG, Thakur AB et al. An integrated approach to the selection of optimal salt form for a new drug candidate. Int J Pharm 1994; 105:209-217.

170. Ross DL, Riley MC. Aqueous solubilities of some variously substituted quinolone antimicrobials. Int J Pharm 1990; 63:237-250.

171. Yalkowsky SH, Banerjee S. Aqueous solubility. New York: Marcel Dekker, 1994.

172. Yalkowsky SH, Valvani SC. Solubility and partitioning I: Solubility of nonelectrolytes in water. J Pharm Sci 1980; 69:912-922.

173. Hafkenscheid TL, Tomlinson E. Isocratic chromatographic retention data for estimating aqueous solubilities of acidic, basic and neutral drugs. Int J Pharm1983; 17:1-21.

174. Nirmalakhandan NN, Speece RE. Quantitative structure-activity relationship models for predicting aqueous solubility. Comparison of three major approaches. ACS Symposium Series 1990; 416:478-485.

175. Nirmalakhandan NN, Speece RE. Prediction of aqueous solubility of organic chemicals based on molecular structure. Environ Sci Technol 1988; 22:328-338.

176. Nirmalakhandan NN, Speece RE. Prediction of aqueous solubility of organic chemicals based on molecular structure. 2. Application the PNAs, PCBs, PCDD, etc. Environ Sci Technol 1989; 23:708-713.

177. Klopman G, Wang S, Balthasar DM. Estimation of aqueous solubility of organic molecules by the group contribution approach. Application of the study of biodegradation. J Chem Inf Comput Sci 1992; 32:474-482.

178. Brüggemann R, Altschuh J. A validation study for the estimation of aqueous solubility from n-octanol/water partition coefficients. The Science of the Total Environment 1991; 109/110:41-57.

179. Nelson TM, Jurs PC. Prediction of aqueous solubility of organic compounds. J Chem Inf Comput Sci 1994; 34:601-609.

180. Suzuki T. Development of an automatic estimation system for both the partition coefficient and aqueous solubility. CHEMICALC-2, Program available from QCPE No. 606, by T. Suzuki. J Comput-Aided Mol Des 1991; 5:149-166.

181. Mitschler LA. The Chemistry of Tetracycline Antibiotics. New York: Marcel Dekker, 1978.

182. Okhamafe AO, Akerele JO, Chukuka CS. Pharmacokinetics of norfloxacin with some metallic medicinal agents. Int J Pharm 1991; 11-18.

183. Ross DL, Elkinton SK, Knaub SR et al. Physicochemical properties of fluoroquinoline antimicrobials. VI Effect of metal-ion complexation on octan-1-ol-water partitioning. Int J Pharm 1993; 93:131-138.

184. Martell AE, Motekaitis RJ. In: Determination and use of stability constants. 2nd ed., New York: VCH, 1992.

185. Rosotti FJC, Rosotti HS. In: The determination of stability constants. New York: McGraw-Hill, 1961: 108.
186. Gans P, Sabatini A, Vacca A. SUPERQUAD: an improved general program for computation of formation constants from potentiometric data. J Chem Soc Dalton Trans 1985:1195-1200.
187. Smith RM, Martell A. Critical Stability Constants, Vol 1-6. New York: Plenum Press, 1974-76, 1982, 1989.

CHAPTER 3

CHEMOMETRIC METHODS USED IN DRUG DISCOVERY

Han van de Waterbeemd

INTRODUCTION

Since the introduction of the concept of quantitative structure-activity relationships (QSAR) in drug discovery in the 1960s and its broad application to the design of biologically active compounds,[1-4] the field has considerably developed.[3-6] New statistical and mathematical methods have been introduced and applied to the design of new molecules and the analysis of chemical and biological data. In the present chapter we deal with the methodology, while examples and applications are found in chapter 4. Our focus is on the most important approaches, including regression and pattern recognition techniques, experimental design, database clustering and validation of the results. The purpose of the chapter is not to explain all methods in full detail, but to give a flavor of current methods and developments. This chapter includes many recent methods of which no or very few successful applications have been reported and therefore should be considered as a status report of present research in this area.

WHY USE CHEMOMETRIC METHODS?

Usually compounds in a drug discovery project are examined in several biological test systems, generating a set of experimental

Structure-Property Correlations in Drug Research, edited by
Han van de Waterbeemd. © 1996 R.G. Landes Company.

data. Typically the data matrix contains missing values, since quite often not all compounds are screened in all available tests. Values for chemical, structural or physicochemical descriptors may be obtained experimentally or be estimated theoretically (chapter 2). The extraction of relevant information from combined biological and chemical data requires appropriate tools. The discipline of chemometrics emerged in the 1970s by work of Wold, Kowalski and Massart. Chemometrics is defined as the application of statistics and mathematics in chemistry,[7] and its history has been summarized by Brereton.[8]

Table 3.1. Overview of chemometric methods used in drug discovery research

Regression / correlation

Multiple linear regression (MLR)[3,26], ordinary least squares (OLS)
Non-linear regression[13]
Partial least squares (PLS)[14-17,24-26,102]
Generating optimal linear PLS estimations (GOLPE)[52]
Adaptive least squares (ALS)[83-85]
Principal components regression (PCR)[27]
Canonical correlation (CC)[28]
Continuum regression (CR)[29]
Ridge regression (RR)
Artificial neural networks (ANN)[30-37,53]
Genetic function algorithm (GFA)[38]
Evolutionary programming (EP)[39,57,58]
Similarity matrices[41-48]
Rule induction[104]

Pattern recognition / classification

Principal component analysis (PCA)[73]
Factor analysis (FA)[73]
Correspondence factor analysis (CFA)[74-77]
Spectral mapping analysis (SMA)[78-81]
Nonlinear mapping (NLM)[5]
Multidimensional scaling (MDS)[47]
Cluster significance analysis (CSA)[64,65]
Cluster analysis (CA)[68-72]
Linear discriminant analysis (LDA)[65,82]
Class analogy (SIMCA)[63]
Linear learning machines (LLM)
k-Nearest neighbours (KNN)[61]
Fuzzy adaptive least squares (FALS)[84,85]
Artificial neural networks (ANN)[30-37,53]
Single class discrimination (SCD)[61,62]

Statistical methods are used in various fields in the pharmaceutical industry, ranging from molecular design and pharmaceutical development,[9] to quality and process control. An overview of various methods used is presented in Table 3.1. Reviews[4,10,11] and recent books[3,5,6] provide good insights into the present status of the field. The classical domain of application entails the development of quantitative structure-activity relationships (QSAR) more broadly in structure-property correlations (SPC) (chapter 1). More recent applications are found in connection to molecular modeling studies, such as three-dimensional QSAR (chapter 5). Finally,

---

Table 3.1. Overview of chemometric methods used in drug discovery research (continued)

Experimental design (for series design, random screening)[86]

CARSO approach[54]
Craig plot[4,89]
Topliss tree[4,88]
Factorial design[87,92, 93]
Fractional factorial design[87,92,93]
D-optimal design[54,93]
Maximum dissimilarity[95]
Cluster sampling[95]
Trend vector analysis[96,97]
Procrustes analysis[94]

Validation[100-103]

Correlation coefficient (r or r[2], adjusted r[2]) for data fitting
Fisher F-test (F)
Standard error of the regression (s)
Jackknife[16]
Bootstrapping[16,102]
Cross-validation (CV): leave-one-out (LOO), leave-groups-out (LGO)[100,101]
Cross-validated correlation coefficient (Q^2) for data prediction[52,54]
Predictive residual sum of squares (PRESS)[52]
Standard deviation of predictions (s_{PRESS})[52]
Standard error of predictions (SDEP)[52,54]
Lack-of-fit (LOF)[38]
Fitness function (FIT)[57,58]
Scrambling of the dependent Y-values[103]

---

the exploration of two- and three-dimensional structure databases, as well as the rational design of combinatorial libraries have become important areas where chemometric approaches are being used. Furthermore, virtual databases, containing modeled rather than experimental structures, may be analyzed. Multivariate statistical methods, such as cluster analysis and similarity-based concepts, are used to exploit the information content of these databases (chapter 6).

REGRESSION TECHNIQUES

MULTIPLE LINEAR REGRESSION (MLR)

Classical quantitative structure-activity relationships (QSAR) or Hansch analysis models derive relationships between biological activity values and physicochemical properties.[1,3] Since, many of the descriptors or parameters used are linear free-energy-related terms, this technique is also called the extrathermodynamic approach. A further well-known method is the Free-Wilson approach,[3,12] using only binary descriptors for presence or absence of particular substructures in the molecule. Equations are mostly computed by either multiple linear regression (MLR), also called ordinary least-squares (OLS), or by non-linear regression. In order to obtain statistically meaningful regression equations, a number of basic requirements have to be fulfilled. These are extensively described in a recent book by Kubinyi.[3] To avoid chance correlations it is important to include only non-collinear parameters in the final equation. A sophisticated treatment of this problem was reported by Mager,[13] who introduced non-least squares (NLS) regression as an alternative to the better known partial least squares (PLS) regression technique, which is discussed below.

PARTIAL LEAST SQUARES (PLS)

Multiple linear regression (MLR) has a number of limitations, which can be dealt with using the partial least squares projection to latent structures (PLS) analysis method.[14,15] Particularly, the ratio of the number of compounds to the number of variables should exceed five in MLR. After initial hesitation of acceptance, the PLS method is now considered as a robust regression and classification technique in structure-property correlation studies.[16] The PLS method is of particular interest in three-dimensional QSAR studies (chapter 5). The underlying NIPALS algorithm designed by H. Wold[17] has been introduced in chemometrics by further developments of Wold[18] and Kowalski.[19] A weakness of normal PLS is that it does not detect nonlinear relationships. Therefore more recent extensions include non-linear[20] and multi-block[21] PLS. Nonlinear relationships can also be detected by using PLS analysis of distance matrices between every compound in the data set.[22] More efficient algorithms to deal with large data sets have been developed, such as the Kernel[23] and SAMPLS[24] algorithm.

COMPARISON OF MLR AND PLS

A number of papers deal with comparisons among regression and correlation methods.[25] Particularly, the performance of PLS has been compared with multiple linear regression,[26] principal components regression (PCR),[27] ridge regression, canonical correlation analysis,[28] and continuum regression.[29] This latter method has been explored by Ford and colleagues as a general regression technique combining the best of MLR, PLS and PCR. These comparative studies give insight as to which method should be used for a particular data set, although in many cases there is no unique answer and a combination of methods seems the best strategy.

ARTIFICIAL NEURAL NETWORKS

Novel pattern recognition technologies are of potential interest to scientists working in the pharmaceutical and related industries. Among these new techniques, artificial neural networks (ANN) had much attention in recent years.[30,31] ANNs are being used in correlation and classification problems, as well as for the prediction of properties such as partition coefficients[32] or aqueous solubility.[33,34]

These network algorithms are an attempt to simulate some of the neurological processing capabilities of the brain. ANNs are parallel information processing systems, which in some applications appear to be superior to the more traditional Von Neumann sequential approach. A neural net can vary in architecture, but in principle is based on a network of processing elements. The most widely applied system is based on the back-propagation network

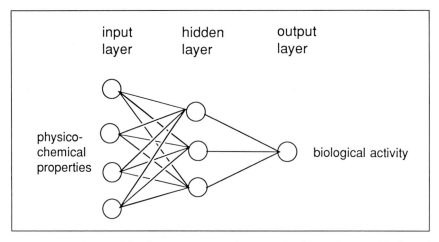

Fig. 3.1. Neural network back–propagation architecture for the prediction of biological activities from physicochemical data input.

(Fig. 3.1). The connections between neurons are given a weight and the network training is performed by varying these weights. The output of a neuron is controlled by a transfer function, for which typically a sigmoidal function is used. Since the weights are adjusted according to the output it is necessary to adjust backwards from the output layer, hence the term back-propagation. Other architectures such as Kohonen topology-preserving mapping have also been tested in drug discovery problems.[35] Another interesting approach is the use of molecular matrices, such as a connectivity or distance matrix, as input and a dynamic network topology.[36]

In principle, ANNs are capable of both selecting important parameters and establishing predictive relationships between them. A strategy has been proposed using selective pruning, cross-validation and ANNs to eliminate all nonrelevant descriptors from a large set.[37] The final set was then used to train back-propagation ANNs to predict biological activity.

GENETIC ALGORITHMS AND EVOLUTIONARY PROGRAMMING

In standard regression approaches, like Hansch analysis, using multiple linear regression, as well as with the PLS method, a single "best" solution is found. However, in many cases almost equivalent solutions based on different combinations of relevant descriptors may exist explaining the dependent biological values equally well. Recently some new methods have been introduced to deal with this problem, including the genetic function algorithm (GFA)[38] and evolutionary programming (EP)[39] method. The GFA has more parameters to be specified by the user than the EP method. Potentially, the EP method finds good quantitative relationships (QSARs) that are missed by the GFA.[39] Therefore, it seems that both methods are complementary. Since these approaches produces sets of solutions, they have been called combinatoric QSAR.

SIMILARITY MATRICES

Methods have been developed to compare the shape and other steric aspects of molecules, as well as their electronic properties. It is assumed that similar molecules exert their biological function through similar modes of action. However, there is no unambigous definition of similarity. Similarity may concern only parts of the molecule, or a global descriptor such as lipophilicity. Various similarity indices have been defined.[40-43] Popular ones are the Carbo and Hodgkin similarity index or the Spearman rank correlation coefficient.[44] Similarities can be collected in a N x N similarity matrix, in which each molecule is compared with all the others in a series. These matrices can be used in QSAR analyses.[45,46] An appropriate tool for the analysis of similarity or dissimilarity matrices is multidimensional scaling.[47] As a typical example it was found that MLP (= molecular lipophilicity potential)-based similarity matrices are capable of distinguishing between properties responsible for dopamine receptor D_1 and D_2 recognition.[48] However, it has been shown that these matrices neither complement the classical QSAR descriptors nor improve their performance.[49]

VARIABLE SELECTION

A priori it is often not evident which variables (descriptors or parameters) are most relevant in a particular situation. Therefore, the strategy generally involves the generation of a large set of descriptors[50,51] and then to use appropriate statistical methods to find the most relevant ones. Traditionally, the most widely used method to find a relevant combination of descriptors was stepwise multiple linear regression. However, this method is not robust, since forward and backward elimination may yield different end results. At present cross-validated PLS[14,15] or the GOLPE[52] approach are considered to be much better choices. A more recent approach is based on artificial neural networks (ANN).[53] The advantage of this latter method is that it implicitly includes nonlinear models, and thus represents a nonlinear regression model in structure-property correlation studies. Some scientists prefer a kind of preprocessing in the selection of descriptors. Indeed, one may first perform a principal component analysis, or cluster analysis, or just have a look at the correlation matrix of all descriptors, and then remove all redundant descriptors.

GOLPE is an advanced PLS technique using D-optimal design variable selection criteria to derive reliable models.[52,54] It has been of particular interest in 3D-QSAR studies (chapter 5) for its efficient handling of large data sets. Validation of the models (see below for further discussion) is performed in GOLPE by leaving groups out in a repeated and random fashion.[54] Another measure for the relative importance of independent variables (also called the x variables) is called VIP (variable influence on the prediction).[54]

Simulated annealing is a computational optimization method that has been used in conformational searching,[55] but which also has been used in statistical problems. Generalized simulated annealing (GSA) has been used in combination with ANN to develop an automated descriptor selection routine.[56] However, the time-consuming calculation is a disadvantage of the method.

Kubinyi[57,58] has proposed an evolutionary algorithm, called MUSEUM (mutation and selection uncover models), for variable selection. It starts from a model containing any number of randomly chosen variables. Random mutation by additions and eliminations of variables leads to new models, which are evaluated by a fitness function. Only the best equation is stored and used for further selection. In contrast to genetic algorithms, cross-over is avoided. It has further been suggested to use a systematic search of all relevant combinations of two and three variables as a preselection and then the evolutionary algorithm to find the best equation.[58]

As already discussed, a promising regression method is based on the genetic algorithm.[38] While many regression techniques result in a single model, the typical feature of using the genetic function approximation (GFA)[38] is that a population of many models is obtained. GFAs may detect nonlinear quantitative relationships.

A well-known data set to illustrate the principles of variable selection is the so-called Selwood data set.[57] This data set contains 31 antifilarial antimycin compounds described by 53 features. Selwood and colleagues used stepwise regression,[59] Wikel and Dow a neural network,[53] McFarland and Gans used cluster significance analysis,[60] Rogers and Hopfinger explored a genetic function algorithm[38] and Kubinyi an evolutionary approach.[57,58] Comparing these methods clearly demonstrates that there is no single unique solution. The models should always be checked on their statistical significance and of course their physicochemical meaning.

PATTERN RECOGNITION
AND CLASSIFICATION METHODS

The recognition of structure or patterns in complex data sets was the prime objective of chemometricians. Among the first tools were cluster analysis methods, which were later expanded to include factor analysis and related methods. Pattern recognition techniques can be subdivided into supervised and unsupervised methods. The objective of the former is to classify a new object (compound) into already predefined classes. The aim of unsupervised methods is to find such an unknown classification.

If a set of active compounds occurs as a cluster within a generally more diffuse cloud of inactives, such a data set is called embedded or asymmetric.[61,62] There are a number of tools to deal with such data sets. These include the SIMCA method,[63] cluster significance analysis (CSA),[64,65] k-nearest neighbor (kNN),[61] single class discrimination (SCD) and its variants,[61,62] the distance-based program EVE,[66] or a discriminant-regression model (DIREM).[67]

CLUSTER ANALYSIS

Cluster analysis (CA) operates on distances in multidimensional property space.[68] In the present context CA can be applied to the clustering of compounds in a drug discovery project, clustering of substituent and molecular properties for experimental design,[4,69] clustering of hits from a database search, and clustering of entire databases.[70,71] There are many different clustering methods. The choice depends on the problem and the available computing power. Among the traditional methods hierarchical agglomerative methods are most used. Well-known are single and complete linkage, centroid and Ward's clustering methods. For the clustering of chemical structures in large databases the Jarvis-Patrick method received much attention[71,72] (see below for further discussion). For the analysis of smaller data sets CA forms a nice complement to other pattern recognition techniques such as principal component analysis or neural networks.

FACTOR ANALYSIS AND PRINCIPAL COMPONENT ANALYSIS

The inspection for correlations and patterns in large multidimensional data tables can only be performed using multivariate methods. Among the widely used methods factor analysis (FA) and principal component analysis (PCA) are best known.[73] Sometimes these two terms are used synonymously. However, factor analysis is the generic term for a family of techniques, including PCA, correspondence analysis, spectral mapping, and nonlinear mapping. Basically in all of these related methods a new set of descriptors is formed by building linear combinations of all variables considered. These new descriptors are called principal components, or latent variables, or principal properties. By plotting these two or three principal components a good idea about clustering and classification in the data is obtained. Of interest are both so-called scores plots (for the compounds) and loadings plots (for the variables). Additional methods such as cluster analysis may help to fine-tune the findings.

CORRESPONDENCE FACTOR ANALYSIS

This technique was developed by Benzécri and other French statisticians.[74,75] Correspondence factor analysis (CFA) is based on the use of χ^2-metrics by looking at a data table as a frequency table. It is assumed that for each cell in the data matrix there is a link between compound i and test result j. As in PCA, a factorial plot reveals the strongest correlations. Although CFA appears to be a powerful method, it is still not widely used. One of the reasons is that interactive computer programs for CFA are not widely available. Good examples of its use can be found in the studies of Gilbert and colleagues,[76] or Doré and coworkers.[77]

SPECTRAL MAPPING

The first paper on spectral mapping analysis (SMA) developed by Lewi appeared in 1976 and deals with the simultaneous analysis of potency and specificity in pharmacological data.[78-80] Characteristic of the method is a specific operation on the data matrix, namely the log double-centering of the pharmacological or biochemical data matrix. This means that in the first step all data are taken in their logarithmic form. Next the mean values are calculated row-by-row, followed by subtraction of these means from all elements in the corresponding rows (this is called row-centering). In SMA this is done for rows and columns (double-centering). The method combines some of the features of PCA and CFA. SMA has been used to identify drug test specifities or the classification of biological activity spectra, but also for the classification of proteins and enzymes, which was called receptor mapping and phylogenetic clustering.[81]

MULTIDIMENSIONAL SCALING

A powerful data reduction method for similarity or dissimilarity matrices is multidimensional scaling (MDS).[47] The algorithm computes coordinates for a set of points in a space such that the distances between pairs of these points fit as closely as possible to measured dissimilarities (or similarities, or indirectly as correlation matrices) between a corresponding set of objects. Missing values are ignored. Although MDS belongs to the family of factor analysis methods, there are some important differences. Often MDS leads to fewer dimensions than PCA. There is also a relation to cluster analysis, since MDS operates on similarity comparable to distances in space.

DISCRIMINANT ANALYSIS

The method of choice for the analysis of discrete biological data in the form of activity ratings (e.g. agonist/antagonist or weak/medium/strong) is often linear discriminant analysis (LDA).[82] Although certainly useful in many cases, curiously often MLR of PLS are the methods of first choice.

ADAPTIVE LEAST SQUARES (ALS)

In order to overcome some shortcomings of LDA, Moriguchi and colleagues developed a new discrimination method called adaptive least squares (ALS).[83-85] More recently this approach was extended as fuzzy adaptive least squares (FALS).[84] Instead of assigning a compound to a single class to build a model with ALS, in FALS compounds may belong to more than one activity class with different degrees of membership. Using this approach, a single equation can be derived, irrespective of the number of different activity classes. Therefore this method is sometimes described as a correlation technique. ALS is used to classify new compounds according to a certain activity level, not to predict an exact value such as a binding constant. Advantages are that only one QSAR equation is obtained and nonlinear dependence of activity can be dealt with. Among the disadvantages should be considered the danger of overfitting.[85]

CLUSTER SIGNIFICANCE ANALYSIS

Like linear discriminant analysis (LDA), cluster significance analysis (CSA) developed by McFarland[64,65] can be used for discrete biological data such agonist-antagonists or active-inactive. The studied variables may be continuous. The difference between LDA and CSA is that LDA requires well-separated data, while CSA can handle embedded data as well.

EXPERIMENTAL DESIGN STRATEGIES

The exploration of property space for new biologically active compounds can be largely improved by a proper experimental design.[86,87] In practice, this is not always straightforward, since highly relevant information on the target may not yet be available. The trend is to design more simple compounds, allowing to synthesize many in parallel. Various strategies have been successfully employed to optimize the design process, as will be discussed below. Compounds should not only be designed for their affinity and selectivity, but other relevant properties related to bioavailability and pharmacokinetics should be considered early. This includes the consideration of constraints for lipophilicity and molecular size in order to optimize membrane permeability. Combinatorial chemistry approaches make these requirements and experimental design techniques of high current interest.[47]

DESIGN OF A SERIES OF COMPOUNDS

If no structural information on the macromolecular target is available, a typical chemical program involves variation of a selected position in a lead compound. The operational schemes proposed by Topliss[88] and the parameter plots by Craig[89] are known to most medicinal chemists as methods for series optimization. In this latter approach substituents can be chosen from a two-dimensional plot of lipophilicity (Fujita-Hansch π values) against electronic properties (Hammett σ values). However, this variation should be performed in more dimensions, taking into account the various physicochemical properties of a substituent, which can be subdivided in lipophilic, steric, electronic/electrostatic and H-bonding properties. An approach to reduce this multidimensional parameter space consists of principal component analysis (PCA).[73] The extracted latent variables or principal components (PC) can be used as new design properties[73] (Fig. 3.2), also called principal properties.[90] A further alternative is to use disjoint principal properties (DPPs), which are based on a separate analysis of sets of substituent properties belonging to a given class, e.g., the class of the property lipophilicity. Advantages and disadvantages of this proposal have been discussed.[90] DPPs are not orthogonal to each other and cannot be used in multiple linear regression (MLR) data modeling, whereas they can be used without problem in PLS modeling.

As shown in Table 3.1, there are a number of more recent techniques which can be used in experimental design of new compounds.[4,87,91] Important ones are factorial design schemes (FDs)[87,92] and D-optimal design.[93] FDs are a simple design concept for a proper sampling of the property space when in a molecule a specific position has to be varied. However, they become impractical when at the same time several positions in a molecule are varied. Then D-optimal designs are more appropriate, particularly when also some constraints, such as excluded volume, have to be considered.[93] In this latter method the determinant of the variance-covariance matrix is calculated. This determinant has a maximum

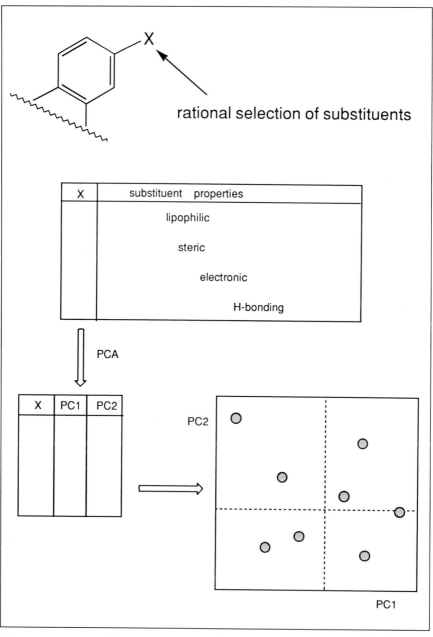

Fig. 3.2. Experimental design for the variation of substituents. Appropriate substituent descriptors for a series of candidate substituents are compiled in a table. Using principal component analysis (PCA) principal properties (PC1 and PC2) are extracted and plotted for making a proper parameter space sampling.

value for those combinations of substituents which have a maximum variance and minimum covariance in their physicochemical descriptors. The variance-covariance matrix is an important cornerstone in matrix operations used in multiple linear regression and principal component analysis, and to obtain a correlation matrix among a set of selected variables.

STRATEGIES FOR RANDOM SCREENING OF COMPOUNDS AND DATABASE CLUSTERING TECHNIQUES

Despite the availability of high throughput screening (HTS), the careful selection of compounds for biological testing remains of great interest in order to use the available amount of sample in the most economic way. A number of strategies based on the clustering of large databases have been proposed to make rational choices.[40,71,94,95] Typical structural descriptors used to perform database clustering include fingerprints (substructural elements), topological indices, calculated physicochemical properties (CLOGP, molecular weight), and indicators for the presence of a hydrophobic group in the molecule. A frequently used measure for similarity between two molecules is the (weighted) Tanimoto index, which is based on substructures and defined as follows:

$$T_{ij} = N_{i\&j} / (N_i + N_j - N_{i\&j})$$

where N_i and N_j are the number of features (substructures) in molecule i and j respectively, and $N_{i\&j}$ the number of common features.

At least two reasons for using experimental design techniques for the selection of compounds for screening can be mentioned:[95] to increase novelty of hits and to improve the hit rate. Two typical strategies have recently been compared using maximum dissimilarity among molecules and cluster sampling techniques like the Jarvis-Patrick method or cluster sampling (CS) based on a nearest neighbor table. However, the performance of these algorithms is rather disappointing.[95] Nevertheless, according to the author,[95] by changing the strategy and using a proper feedback on the testing, a substantial increase in hit rate can be obtained. A further method for the ranking of large collections of chemical compounds is trend vector analysis.[96] A trend vector is defined as a one-dimensional array of correlations between a biological activity and a set of descriptors. Recently the method has been extended[97] using a new formulation of the partial least squares (PLS) method named SAMPLS[24] to handle the large data matrices more efficiently. The approach has two potential applications. One is to select compounds from a database of existing compounds for submission to random screening. The other is the evaluation of chemical structures from a virtual library of candidates for synthesis, which will be discussed next in more detail.

RATIONAL DESIGN OF COMBINATORIAL LIBRARIES

An increasingly important new technology for lead finding is the synthesis and rapid automatic screening on activity as well as absorption potential of combinatorial mixtures of compounds. A rational design of such libraries of compounds would further optimize the discovery process. Critical is the selection of relevant descriptors to define diversity in the library and at the same time to consider bioavailability properties of the compounds. An example of this approach is the study by Martin and colleagues.[47] Obviously, the molecular size should not be too high since high molecular weights limit oral absorption. Furthermore, for oral absorption or uptake in the brain optimal lipophilicity ranges can be defined, which should be part of the design. Descriptors have been proposed characterizing lipophilicity, shape, degree of branching, chemical functionality, specific binding features.[47] It was also demonstrated that a combination of multidimensional scaling (MDS) and D-optimal design[93] has advantages over cluster analysis and selecting one or more compounds from a cluster. However, cluster analysis has the advantage that it can handle much larger data sets. A statistical technique called procrustes analysis followed by PCA has been suggested to analyze different property sets characterizing a diverse set of compounds.[94] This is important to define the most appropriate variables to describe similarity within a compound set. Methods will have to be developed to quantify differences in diversity between libraries and between large databases, in order to evaluate the added value of a new library to the existing database.

GENETIC ALGORITHMS IN SERIES DESIGN

Genetic algorithms (GA) are very efficient computational methods for exploring large combinatorial spaces. They are based on Darwinian principles of evolution. Entities are represented as a "genome," a linear set of genes. Each gene may have one or a set of values, called an "allele." Beginning with a start population, new generations are constructed through mechanisms of selection, mutation and cross-over. Since genetic algorithms are stochastic, random selection is involved at each step. It should be noted that different protocols may be followed.

Sheridan and Kearsley[98] used GA to find a subset of fragments frequently occurring in compounds with the desired pharmacological or biochemical profile. The GA used was based on scoring by two topological methods, namely similarity probes and trend vectors. Topological scoring functions are computationally fast, but have limitations for flexibility and stereochemistry. Automated generation of molecules within constraints using a GA may lead to compounds which cannot easily be synthesized. However, these molecules may be used to construct a pharmacophore (also called biohypothesis) for searching in 3D databases.[99]

VALIDATION OF MODELS

An important aspect of statistical approaches is the validation of the result.[100-103] Any model should not only be statistically sound, but should also make physicochemical sense and have real predictive value. Traditional approaches to judge the quality of a model, originating from linear regression methods, is the correlation coefficient r, characterizing the overall fit. Modern tools for validation include cross-validation and bootstrapping,[102] and scrambling of the dependent variable.[103]

In cross-validation the data set is divided into groups. One group is left out, and a new model is computed and the left-out group predicted. This is repeated a number of times until all compounds have been left out once. The total sum of squares of predictions minus observations is called PRESS, and is a measure of the predictive power of the model. From PRESS two other values can be calculated, which are used to validate the model. $SDEP = (PRESS/n)^{1/2}$ and $Q^2 = 1 - PRESS/SSY$, where SSY is the sum of squares of observations minus mean. This latter Q^2 is also called the cross-validated correlation coefficient (also written as r^2_{cv}) and should be > 0.3. Much debate is still ongoing on the leave-one-out (LOO) cross-validation procedure. Some believe that a better approach is the leave-several-out approach, where about seven groups are optimal.[101] The LOO method has the advantage that it gives reproducible results, whereas by leaving out groups the cross-

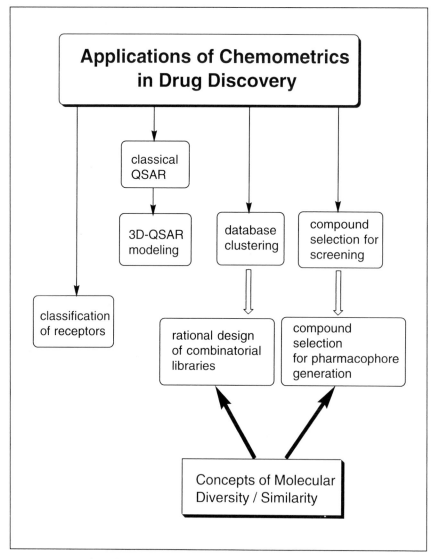

Fig. 3.3. Potential applications of molecular similarity concepts.

validated correlation coefficient varies from one run to another. Statistical evaluation of more recent methods is still an ongoing debate. For example, the results of an evolutionary algorithm as used in the MUSEUM approach[55,56] can be evaluated by a fitness function. Several proposals have been made, including the lack-of-fit (LOF),[38] FIT value[57] and s_{PRESS}.[57] Further investigations are warranted.

The best validation of the discussed methods is their practical use in drug research. For many of the newer approaches none or only a few applications have been reported. Therefore, a final judgment is premature at the present time. Typical applications and more discussions on some of the critical issues are found in chapter 4.

REFERENCES

1. Hansch C, Leo A. Exploring QSAR. Washington: ACS, 1995.
2. Hansch C, Sammes PG, Taylor JB, eds. Comprehensive Medicinal Chemistry, Vol 4. Quantitative Drug Design. Oxford: Pergamon Press, 1990.
3. Kubinyi H. QSAR: Hansch Analysis and Related Approaches. Weinheim: VCH, 1993.
4. van de Waterbeemd H. Quantitative approaches to structure-activity relationships. In: Wermuth CG, ed. The Practice of Medicinal Chemistry. London: Academic Press, 1995.
5. van de Waterbeemd H, ed. Chemometric Methods in Molecular Design. Weinheim: VCH, 1995.
6. van de Waterbeemd H, ed. Advanced Computer-Assisted Techniques in Drug Discovery. Weinheim: VCH, 1994.
7. Massart DL, Vandeginste BGM, Deming SN et al. Chemometrics: a Textbook. Amsterdam: Elsevier, 1988.
8. Brereton R. Chemometrics. Applications of Mathematics and Statistics to Laboratory Systems. New York: Ellis Horwood, 1995.
9. Lindberg NO, Lundstedt T. Application of multivariate analysis in pharmaceutical development work. Drug Dev Ind Pharm 1995; 21:987-1007.
10. Stone M, Jonathan P. Statistical thinking and technique for QSAR and related studies. Part I: General theory. J Chemom 1993; 7:455-475.
11. Stone M, Jonathan P. Statistical thinking and technique for QSAR and related studies. Part II: Specific methods. J Chemom 1994; 8:1-20.

12. Free SM, Wilson JW. A mathematical contribution to structure-activity studies. J Med Chem 1964; 7:395-399.

13. Mager PP. Non-least-squares regression analysis applied to organic and medicinal chemistry. Med Chem Revs 1994; 14:533-588.

14. Wold S, Johansson E, Cocchi M. PLS—partial least-squares projections to latent strucures. In: Kubinyi H, ed. 3D QSAR in Drug Design. Leiden: ESCOM, 1993:523-550.

15. Wold S. PLS for multivariate linear modeling. In: van de Waterbeemd H, ed. Chemometric Methods in Molecular Design. Weinheim: VCH, 1995:195-218.

16. Hansson LO, Waters N, Holm S et al. On the quantitative structure-activity relationships of meta-substituted (S)-phenylpiperidines, a class of preferential dopamine D_2 autoreceptor ligands: modeling of dopamine synthesis and relase in vivo by means of partial least squares regression. J Med Chem 1995; 38:3121-3131.

17. Wold H. Soft modeling by latent variables: the nonlinear iterative partial least squares (NIPALS) algorithm. In: Gani J, ed. Perspectives in Probability and Statistics. London: Academic Press, 1975:117-142.

18. Wold S, Albano C, Dunn III WJ et al. Pattern recognition: finding and using patterns in multivariate data. In: Martens H, Russwurm Jr H, eds. Food Research and Data Analysis. London: Applied Science Publ, 1983:147-188.

19. Gerlach RW, Kowalski BR, Wold H, Partial least-squares path modeling with latent variables. Anal Chim Acta 1979; 112:417-421.

20. Wold S, Kettaneh-Wold N, Skagerberg B. Nonlinear PLS modelling. Chemometr Intell Lab Syst 1989; 7:53-65.

21. Wangen LE, Kowalski BR. A multiblock partial least squares algorithm for investigating complex chemical systems. J Chemometr 1988; 3:3-20.

22. Martin YC, Lin CT, Hetti C et al. PLS analysis of distance matrices to detect nonlinear relationships between biological potency and molecular properties. J Med Chem 1995; 38:3009-3015.

23. Lindgren F, Geladi P, Wold S. The kernel algorithm for PLS. J Chemometr 1993; 7:45-49.

24. Bush BL, Nachbar RB. Sample-distance partial least squares: PLS optimized for many variables, with application to CoMFA. J Comp Aid Mol Des 1993; 7:587-619.

25. Frank IE, Friedman JH. A statistical view of some chemometric regression tools. Technometr 1993; 35:109-148.

26. Verhaar HJM, Eriksson L, Sjöström M et al. Modelling the toxicity of organophosphates: a comparison of the multiple linear regression and PLS regression methods. Quant Struct-Act Relat 1994; 13:133-143.

27. De Jong S. PLS fits closer than PCR. J Chemometr 1993; 7:551-557.

28. Ford MG, Salt DW. The use of canonical correlation analysis. In: van de Waterbeemd H, ed. Chemometric Methods in Molecular Design. Weinheim: VCH, 1995:265-282.

29. Malpass JA, Salt DW, Ford MG et al. Continuum regression: a new algorithm for the prediction of biological activity. In: van de Waterbeemd H, ed. Advanced Computer-Assisted Techniques in Drug Discovery. Weinheim: VCH, 1995:163-189.

30. Achanta AS, Kowalski JG, Rhodes CT. Artificial neural networks: implications for pharmaceutical sciences. Drug Dev Ind Pharm 1995; 21:119-155.

31. Zupan J, Gasteiger J. Neural Networks for Chemists. Weinheim: VCH, 1993.

32. Cense JM, Diawara B, Legendre JJ et al. Neural networks prediction of partition coefficients. Chemom Intell Lab Syst 1994; 23:301-308.

33. Bodor N, Harget A, Huang MJ. Neural network studies I. Estimation of the aqueous solubility of organic compounds. J Am Chem Soc 1991; 113:9480-9483.

34. Chow H, Chen H, Ng T et al. Using backpropagation networks for the estimation of aqueous activity coefficients of aromatic organic compounds. J Chem Inf Comput Sci 1995; 35:723-728.

35. Rose VS, Croall IF, MacFie HJH. An application of unsupervised neural network methodology (Kohonen topology-preserving mapping) to QSAR analysis. Quant Struct Act Relat 1991; 10:6-15.

36. Kireev DB. ChemNet: a novel neural network based method for graph/property mapping. J Chem Inf Comput Sci 1995; 35:175-180.

37. Maddelena DJ, Johnston GAR. Prediction of receptor properties and binding affinity of ligands to benzodiazepine/GABA$_A$ receptors using artificial neural networks. J Med Chem 1995; 38:717-724.

38. Rogers D, Hopfinger AJ. Application of genetic function approximation to quantitative structure-activity relationships and quantitative structure- property relationships. J Chem Inf Comput Sci 1994; 34:854-866.

39. Luke BT. Evolutionary programming applied to the development of quantitative structure-activity relationships and quantitative structure-property relationships. J Chem Inf Comput Sci 1994; 34:1279-1287.

40. Johnson MA, Maggiora GM, Lajiness MS et al. Molecular similarity analysis: applications in drug discovery. In: van de Waterbeemd H, ed. Advanced Computer-Assisted Techniques in Drug Discovery. Weinheim: VCH, 1995:89-110.

41. Burt C. Molecular similarity calculations for the rational design of bioactive molecules. In: Vinter JG, Gardner M, eds. Molecular Modeling and Drug Design. London: Macmillan, 1994:305-332.

42. Good AC. The calculation of molecular similarity: alternative formulas, data manipulation and graphical display. J Mol Graphics 1992; 10:144-151.

43. Good AC, Richards WG. Rapid evaluation of shape similarity using Gaussian functions. J Chem Inf Comp Sci 1993; 33:112-116.

44. Sanz F, Manaut F, Rodriguez J et al. A computational package for analysis and comparison of molecular electronic potentials. J Comput Aided Mol Des 1993; 7:337.

45. Good AC, So S-S, Richards WG. Structure-activity relationships from molecular similarity matrices. J Med Chem 1993; 36:433-438.

46. Good AC, Peterson SJ, Richards WG. QSAR's from similarity matrices. Technique validation and application in the comparison of different similarity evaluation methods. J Med Chem 1993; 36:2929-2937.

47. Martin EJ, Blaney JM, Siani MA et al. Measuring diversity: experimental design of combinatorial libraries for drug discovery. J Med Chem 1995; 38:1431-1436.

48. Bone RGA, Villar HO. Discriminating D1 and D2 agonists with a hydrophobic similarity index. J Mol Graph 1995; 13:201-208.

49. Benigni R, Cotta-Ramusino A, Giorgio F et al. Molecular similarity matrices and quantitative structure-activity relationships: a case study with methodological implications. J Med Chem 1995; 38:629-635.

50. van de Waterbeemd H, Testa B. The parametrization of lipophilicity and other structural properties in drug design. Adv Drug Res 1987; 16:85-225.

51. Murugan R, Grendze MP, Toomey Jr JE. Predicting physical properties from molecular structure. Chemtech 1994; June:17-23.

52. Baroni M, Costantino G, Cruciani G et al. Generating optimal linear PLS estimations (GOLPE): an advanced chemometric tool for handling 3D- QSAR problems. Quant Struct Act Relat 1993; 12:9-20.

53. Wikel J, Dow E. The use of neural networks for variable selection in QSAR. Bioorg Med Chem Lett 1993; 3:645-651.

54. Clementi S, Cruciani G, Riganelli D et al. Modelling and chemometrics in medicinal chemistry. In: Dean PM, Jolles G, Newton CG, eds. New Perspectives in Drug Design. London: Academic Press, 1995:285-310.

55. Wilson SR, Cui W. Conformation searching using simulated annealing. In: Merz K, Le Grand S, eds. The Protein Folding Problem and Tertiary Structure Prediction. Boston: Birkhäuser, 1994.

56. Sutter JM, Dixon SL, Jurs PC. Automated descriptor selection for quantitative structure-activity relationships using generalized simulated annealing. J Chem Inf Comput Sci 1995; 35:77-84.

57. Kubinyi H. Variable selection in QSAR studies. I. An evolutionary algorithm. Quant Struct-Act Relat 1994; 13:285-294.

58. Kubinyi H. Variable selection in QSAR studies. II. A highly efficient combination of systematic search and evolution. Quant Struct-Act Relat 1994; 13:393-401.

59. Selwood DL, Livingstone DJ, Comley JCW et al. Structure-activity relationship of antifilarial antimycin analogues: a multivariate pattern recognition study. J Med Chem 1990; 33:136-142.

60. McFarland JW, Gans DJ. On identifying likely determinants of biological activity in high dimensional QSAR problems. Quant Struct Act Relat 1994; 13:11-17.

61. Rose VS, Wood J, MacFie HJH. Analysis of embedded data: k-nearest neighbor and single class discrimination. In: van de Waterbeemd H, ed. Advanced Computer-Assisted Techniques in Drug Discovery. Weinheim: VCH, 1995:228-243.

62. Rose VS, Wood J, MacFie HJH. Single class discrimination using principal component analysis (SCD-PCA). Quant Struct Act Relat 1991; 10:359-368.

63. Wold S. Pattern recognition by means of disjoint principal components models. Pattern Recog 1976; 8:127-139.

64. McFarland JW, Gans DJ. Cluster significance analysis contrasted with three other quantitative structure-activity relationship models. J Med Chem 1987; 30:46-49.

65. McFarland JW. Linear discriminant analysis and cluster significance analysis. In: Hansch C, Sammes PG, Taylor JB, eds. Comprehensive Medicinal Chemistry, Vol 4. Quantitative Drug Design. Oxford: Pergamon Press, 1990:667-689.

66. Benigni R. EVE, a distance based approach for discriminating nonlinearly separable groups. Quant Struct-Act Relat 1994; 13:406-411.

67. Raevsky O, Sapegin A, Zefirov N. The QSAR discriminant-regression model. Quant Struct-Act Relat 1994; 13:412-418.

68. Bratchell N. Cluster analysis. Chemom Intell Lab Syst 1989; 6:105-125.

69. van de Waterbeemd H, El Tayar N, Carrupt PA et al. Pattern recognition study of QSAR substituent descriptors. J Comput Aided Mol Des 1989; 3:111-132.

70. Downs GM, Willett P. Similarity searching and clustering of chemical structure databases using molecular property data. J Chem Inf Comput Sci 1994; 34:1094-1102.

71. Downs GM, Willett P. Clustering of chemical structure databases for compound selection. In: van de Waterbeemd H, ed. Advanced Computer-Assisted Techniques in Drug Discovery. Weinheim: VCH, 1995:111-130.

72. Jarvis RA, Patrick EA. IEEE Trans Comput 1973; C-22:1025-1034.

73. Franke R, Gruska A. Multivariate data analysis of chemical and biological data. In: van de Waterbeemd H, ed. Chemometric Methods in Molecular Design. Weinheim: VCH, 1995:113-164.

74. Greenacre MJ. Theory and Application of Correspondence Analysis. London: Academic Press, 1984.

75. Doré JC, Ojasoo T. Molecular taxonomy by correspondence factorial analysis. In: van de Waterbeemd H, ed. Advanced Computer-Assisted Techniques in Drug Discovery. Weinheim: VCH, 1995:190-227.

76. Gilbert J, Doré J-C, Bignon E et al. Study of the effects of basic di- and tri-phenyl derivatives on malignant cell profileration: an example of the application of correspondence factor analysis to structure-activity relationships (SAR). Quant Struc-Act Relat 1994; 13:262-274.

77. Ojasoo T, Raynaud JP, Doré JC. Correspondence factor analysis of steroid libraries. Steroids 1995; 60:458-469.

78. Lewi PJ. Spectral mapping, a technique for classifying biological activity profiles of chemical compounds. Arzeim Forsch 1976; 26:1295-1300.

79. Lewi PJ, Analysis of biological activity profiles by Spectramap. Eur J Med Chem 1986; 21:155-162.

80. Lewi PJ. Spectral map analysis: factorial analysis of contrasts, especially from log ratios. Chem Int Lab Syst 1989; 5:105-116.

81. Lewi PJ, Moereels, H. Receptor mapping and phylogenetic clustering. In: van de Waterbeemd H, ed. Advanced Computer-Assisted Techniques in Drug Discovery. Weinheim: VCH, 1995:131-162.

82. van de Waterbeemd H. Discriminant analysis for activity prediction. In: van de Waterbeemd H, ed. Chemometric Methods in Molecular Design. Weinheim: VCH, 1995:283-293.

83. Moriguchi I, Komatsu K, Matsushita Y. Adaptive least-squares method applied to structure-activity correlation of hypotensive N-alkyl-N''-cyano- N'-pyridylguanidines. J Med Chem 1980; 23:20-26.

84. Moriguchi I, Hirono S, Liu Q et al. Fuzzy adaptive least squares and its use in quantitative structure-activity relationships. Chem Pharm Bull 1990; 38:3373-3379.

85. Schaper KJ. Quantitative analysis of structure-activity-class relationships by (fuzzy) adaptive least squares. In: van de Waterbeemd H, ed. Advanced Computer-Assisted Techniques in Drug Discovery. Weinheim: VCH, 1995:244-280.

86. Goupy JL. Methods for Experimental Design. Amsterdam: Elsevier, 1993.

87. Austel V. Experimental design in synthesis planning and structure-property correlations. In: van de Waterbeemd H, ed. Chemometric Methods in Molecular Design. Weinheim: VCH, 1995:49-62.

88. Topliss JG. Utilization of operational schemes for analog synthesis in drug design. J Med Chem 1972; 15:1006-1011.

89. Craig P. Interdependence between physical paramters and selection of substituent groups for correlation studies. J Med Chem 1971; 14:680-684.

90. van de Waterbeemd H, Costantino G, Clementi S et al. Disjoint principal properties of organic substituents. In: van de Waterbeemd H, ed. Chemometric Methods in Molecular Design. Weinheim: VCH, 1995:103-112.

91. Sjöström M, Eriksson L. Applications of statistical design and PLS modeling in QSAR. In: van de Waterbeemd H, ed. Chemometric Methods in Molecular Design. Weinheim: VCH, 1995:63-90.

92. Pastor M, Alvarez-Builla J. The EDISFAR programs. Drug series design in polysubstituted prototypes. Quant Struct-Act Relat 1995; 14:24-30.

93. Baroni M, Clementi S, Cruciani G. D-optimal designs in QSAR. Quant Struct Act Relat 1993; 12:225-231.

94. Rose VS, Rahr E, Hudson BD. The use of procrustes analysis to compare different property sets for the characterization of a diverse set of compounds. Quant Struct Act Relat 1994; 13:152-158.

95. Taylor R. Simulation analysis of experimental design strategies for screening random compounds as potential new drugs and agrochemicals. J Chem Inf Comput Sci 1995; 35:59-67.

96. Carhart RE, Smith DH, Venkataghavan R. Atom pairs as molecular features in structure-activity studies: Definition and application. J Chem Inf Compu Sci 1985; 25:64-73.

97. Sheridan RP, Nachbar RB, Bush BL. Extending the trend vector: the trend matrix and sample-based partial least squares. J Compt Aid Mol Des 1994; 8:323-340.

98. Sheridan RP, Kearsley SK. Using a genetic algorithm to suggest combinatorial libraries. J Chem Inf Comput Sci 1995; 35:310-320.

99. Glen RC, Payne AWR. A genetic algorithm for the automated generation of molecules within constraints. J Comput Aid Mol Des 1995; 9:181-202.

100. Wold S. Validation of QSAR's. Quant Struct Act Relat 1991; 10:191-193.

101. Clementi S, Wold S. How to choose the proper statistical method. In: van de Waterbeemd H, ed. Chemometric Methods in Molecular Design. Weinheim: VCH, 1995:319-338.

102. Cramer III RD, Bunce JD, Patterson DE et al. Crossvalidation, bootstrapping, and partial least squares compared with multiple regression in conventional QSAR studies. Quant Struct Act Relat 1988; 7:18-25.
103. Klopman G, Kalos AN. Causality in structure-activity studies. J Comp Chem 1985; 5:492-506.
104. A-Razzak M, Glen RC. Rule induction applied to the derivation of quantitative structure-activity relationships. In: van de Waterbeemd H, ed. Advanced Computer-Assisted Techniques in Drug Discovery. Weinheim: VCH, 1995:319-331.

CHAPTER 4

STRUCTURE PROPERTY CORRELATIONS IN MOLECULAR DESIGN

David J. Livingstone

INTRODUCTION

Other chapters in this book have shown how chemical structures may be characterized by physicochemical properties—measured, predicted, calculated and theoretical, and how a wide variety of mathematical and statistical methods may be used to examine relationships between some desired property of interest, such as biological activity, and these descriptors. The purpose of this chapter is to illustrate by example the application of these techniques and, in particular, to show the diversity of both the methods and the types of property which can predicted or modeled. Before showing modern examples of the use of structure-property correlations (SPC), however, it is instructive to consider one of the earliest[*] publications in this field.[1] Crum Brown and Fraser wrote an equation in which physiological action, F, was related to a function of "chemical constitution," C, thus:

$$\Phi = f(C) \tag{1}$$

---

[*] *Other authors sometimes cite earlier examples, for instance Blake, Am J Med Sci, 1851, but this paper by Crum Brown and Frazer is still relevant today.*

Structure-Property Correlations in Drug Research, edited by Han van de Waterbeemd. © 1996 R.G. Landes Company.

In their report it was acknowledged that it was not possible to obtain an accurate mathematical definition of f in Equation 1 because it was not possible to express changes in the chemical constitution (ΔC) with sufficient "definiteness." Despite the large amount of effort that has gone into research into the characterization of chemical structure in terms of physicochemical properties, this statement probably holds true today. A recent report on the creation of quantitative structure-property relationships identifies some 400 molecular descriptors which can be used to define molecules and discusses the problem of the recognition of the most appropriate ones.[2] The following examples have been chosen from the recent literature (since 1990); for a wider perspective there are a number of useful reviews, specialist publications and proceedings of meetings.[3-8] They have been organized in terms of the main analytical method used to construct them, with the exception of the section on chemical property predictions. They could, of course, have been organized by activity or disease type but, hopefully, this division will keep the examples within a reasonable number of sensible divisions.

REGRESSION MODELS

Regression analysis was one of the first techniques used to create SPCs and although other techniques such as pattern recognition are becoming more widely used,[9] regression remains the most popular. An example of a quite "classical" regression model, involving solely partition coefficient as the physicochemical descriptor, is shown in Equation 2:[10]

$$\log 1/C = 0.41(\pm 0.13) \log P + 1.99(\pm 0.83) \tag{2}$$

$$n = 16 \quad r = 0.88 \quad s = 0.126 \quad F = 48.8$$

The C in this equation is the minimum concentration for inhibition of growth of the fungus *C. albicans* by a set of substituted 1,5-diarylpyrroles. Figures in brackets are the standard errors for the coefficients and the statistics of fit for the model are given below the equation. The inclusion of a hydrophobicity term, whether as log P, π, chromatographic retention or some calculated quantity, is very common in regression models of biological data; indeed, in a survey of relationships abstracted by the journal

Quantitative Structure-Activity Relationships and reported in the journal itself for 1988 over 40% involved a hydrophobicity related parameter.[3] Of course the other physicochemical descriptors proposed in the early Hansch papers[11] may also be found in current applications:[12]

$$\log (1/\text{MIC}) = 0.87(\pm 0.27)\sigma - 0.88(\pm 0.19)I_4 - \qquad (3)$$
$$0.017(\pm 0.007)MW + 5.39(\pm 2.48)$$

$$n = 30 \quad r = 0.92 \quad s = 0.23 \quad F = 47.8 \quad r^2_{cv} = 0.79$$

This equation relates the minimum inhibitory concentration (MIC) of a series of sulphanilamido-1-phenylpyrazoles against whole *E. coli* cells to σ and molecular weight (MW). Once again, the statistics for the fit of the model are shown below the equation and in this case an extra statistic, r^2_{cv}, is reported which is a measure of the predictive power* of the equation. The second term in the equation, I_4, is an indicator variable which codes for substitution type, taking a value of 1 for one sub-series and 0 for another. This is quite a common means by which different but related subsets of compounds may be combined into the same regression equation, or any other quantitative model for that matter. There is, however, one potential problem with the use of indicator variables in regression modeling. The indicator serves to shift the line (or plane for a multidimensional case) for one of the subsets so that it becomes coincident with the line for the other subset. If the two lines have the same slope, or in the case of hyperplanes the same general orientation, then all is well and the indicator will produce a larger, homogeneous set. If, however, the slopes of the two lines are different, then use of the indicator variable will produce a new model which does not correctly fit either of the subsets. The situation may be easily checked for a single indicator variable by fitting individual equations to the two subsets and checking that the regression coefficients of the separate models are similar. But where multiple indicator variables are used (a quite common situation) it is much more difficult to avoid such problems.

---

* *This is the correlation coefficient of a plot of predicted vs. observed values where predictions were made by the leave-one-out method.*

There are numerous examples of published relationships involving substituent constant data such as π, σ and MR, and doubtless many unpublished ones too, but there is one major drawback to this approach and that is the availability of suitable tabulated data. When the compounds of interest all belong to a closely related series then it is usually possible to characterize them fairly adequately using literature data. But when, for example, the only common element is an amide group, as a recently published example shows,[13] it is not possible to use this approach. One solution to this problem is to use descriptors such as molecular connectivity indices which are based solely on the molecular structure, e.g., bonds, atoms, fragments, paths etc. It is claimed that models based on these topological or "non-empirical" descriptors are "emerging as the method of choice"[14] although the physicochemical significance of these descriptors has been questioned.[15] An alternative is to create computer models of the molecules and "measure" or calculate descriptors such as molecular dimensions and electronic distributions from the models.[16-20] An example of a correlation involving such descriptors for a set of compounds which induce α-2μ-globulin nephropathy[21] is shown in Equation 4:

$$\log IC_{50} = 4.5(\pm 1.5)Q^- - 0.044(\pm 0.008)MV + 2.5 \qquad (4)$$

$$n = 12 \quad r^2 = 0.84 \quad s = 0.53 \quad r^2_{cv} = 0.6$$

Here the IC_{50} values are binding affinities to α-2μ-globulin measured by displacement of tritiated 2,2,4-trimethylpentan-2-ol from male rat kidney cytosol. The two descriptors in the equation, Q^- (for the most electronegative atom) and molar volume (MV), may be calculated for any molecule and thus, in principle, this relationship is "generic" and may be used to make a prediction for any molecule.*

An alternative approach to the use of generalized molecular parameters such as molar volume is to calculate descriptors based on some specific molecular features (see also the section on 3D-QSAR). An example of a correlation between 5HT$_{1A}$ receptor binding and a size-shape descriptor[22] (see reference for full details) is shown in Figure 4.1 and Equation 5.

---

* *A relationship such as this, of course, only holds for compounds which are "similar" to the training set although a definition of similarity may be problematical.*

$$pA(5HT_{1A}) = 8.0(\pm 1.0)\,VD(norm)(5HT_{1A}) + 4.5(\pm 0.4) \qquad (5)$$

$$n = 18 \quad r = 0.902 \quad s = 0.724 \quad F = 65.27$$

The size-shape descriptor was calculated for each ligand by reference to a "supermolecule" created by the superimposition of the four most active and structurally dissimilar ligands in the set. Hopfinger and Kawakami have similarly reported[23] a highly specific QSAR for a set of anti-cancer benzothiopyranoindazole derivatives:

$$-\log(IC_{50}) = -0.46(\pm 0.02)[E + \Delta E_D] - 0.46 \qquad (6)$$
$$n = 14 \quad r = 0.97 \quad s = 0.13$$

The physicochemical descriptors in this equation are a free-space intercalation binding energy (E) and an aqueous desolvation energy (ΔE_D) based on molecular dynamics simulations. Thus, not only is it possible to calculate physicochemical parameters based on "static" computer models of molecules, it is also possible to take into account conformational flexibility.[24]

It is easy to think that the use of computational chemistry in this way is a particularly modern phenomenon but in fact this is not the case. Yoneda and Nitta published[25] a relationship between

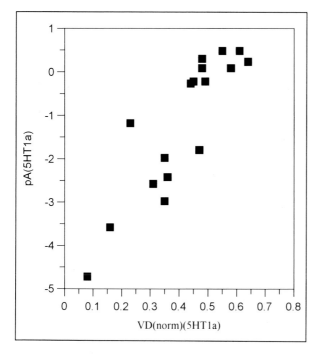

Fig. 4.1. Plot of experimental 5HT_{1A} receptor binding against the ad hoc size-shape descriptor $V_D(norm)$ (5HT_{1A}). (Reproduced with permission from De Benedetti PG, Cocchi M, Menziani MC et al. J Mol Struct (Theochem) 1994; 305:101-10. © 1994 Elsevier Science.)

Table 4.1. Some recently published examples of descriptors calculated by computational chemistry techniques

Description	Symbol	Ref.
Conformational energy (steric) and (electronic)	Jm_n and JS_n	26
Electrostatic potential and shape chirality coefficients	R_{AB}' and S_{AB}'	27
Energy of highest occupied molecular orbital	E_{HOMO}	28
Energy of lowest unoccupied molecular orbital	E_{LUMO}	29
Conformational entropy	S	30
Intrinsic molecular shape and molecular field tensors	$V_u(s,\alpha,\beta)$ Fu $(p,r_{i,j,k},f,\alpha,\beta)$	31
Nucleophilic superdelocalisability	SN_{LUMO}	20
Charge-transfer interaction	CT	32
Surface tension	S	30
Atomic charge	$C(n)$	33
Dipole moment	C_DIPMOM	34

antibacterial activity and nucleophilic superdelocalizability in 1964, about the same time as the (now traditional) Hansch approach was being suggested. Many different properties have been calculated from molecular modeling packages. Table 4.1 shows a few examples of recently published descriptors and reference 3 gives further examples of calculated, particularly electronic, properties.

The combination of computational chemistry and QSAR shows that these two methods which were often thought of as "competitors" are in fact quite complementary and are simply different "tools" in the molecular designers toolbox. Molecular modeling, however, has another function in that it can be used to check the "reasonableness" of correlation equations. There is no reason why a regression model (or any other model for that matter) should have any "causal" foundation but it is comforting to think that at least in some circumstances they do. Quite fittingly, Hansch has shown a number of examples where molecular graphics "pictures" may be used to "explain" QSAR models.[35]

PRINCIPAL COMPONENTS AND RELATED METHODS

Partial least squares (PLS), a relation of principal component regression, is probably the next most popular method in QSAR after regression, although many applications involve "3D-QSAR" (see later section in this chapter). A good example of the use of PLS and also a comparison with Multiple Linear Regression (MLR) was reported by Bordi and coworkers.[36] This study involved a set of histamine H_3 receptor antagonists described by both measured (HPLC capacity factors) and tabulated substituent constants (π, σ, MR, F, R and Verloop Sterimol parameters). A PLS model containing one latent variable was fitted to a set of eight compounds, giving the cross-validated predictions shown in Figure 4.2. This latent variable was composed of both bulk (MR, L and B_5 had high loadings) and lipophilicity and explained ~95% of the variance in the receptor binding data and ~45% of the variance in the descriptor data. A second latent variable, composed mostly of the electronic parameters, explained a further 30% of the variance in the descriptors but only ~1.5% of the biological variance and thus was not considered useful. A plot of pIC_{50} values calculated by the PLS model against the observed values gave a very good straight line but the leave-one-out cross-validated predictions gave the expected somewhat worse fit as shown in Figure 4.2. The major failure of this model is in the prediction for the most active compound, 4a, which suggests that it will be least reliable in prediction

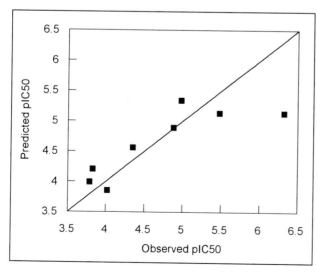

Fig. 4.2. Plot of predicted vs observed pIC_{50} data. Predictions were made from a one component PLS model by leave-one-out cross-validation. (Reproduced with permission from Bordi F, et al. Il Farmaco 1994; 49:153-66. © 1994 Societa Chimica Italiana).

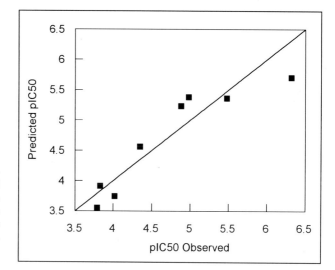

Fig. 4.3. Plot of predicted vs observed pIC_{50} data. Predictions were made from Equation 7 by leave-one-out cross-validation.

for the most active compounds. A number of significant two and three variable multiple linear regression models were fitted to these data. Like the PLS model, these equations contained both bulk and lipophilicity terms and one such model containing an experimental HPLC capacity factor and substituent maximum width is shown in Equation 7:

$$pIC_{50} = -1.098(\pm 0.37) \log k - 0.37(\pm 0.07)B5 + 6.85(\pm 0.29) \quad (7)$$

$$n = 8 \quad r^2 = 0.935 \quad s = 0.269 \quad F = 35.8$$

Leave-one-out cross-validated predictions are shown in Figure 4.3 where it can be seen that this regression model does at least as well if not better than the somewhat more complicated (four variables with "high" loadings) PLS model. It is encouraging that both of these methods give similar results for this data set and, of course, it is a matter of taste as to which technique, if any, is to be preferred. The failure of both models to adequately forecast the activity of compound 4a suggests that the chosen starting variables do not contain sufficient relevant information to model all of the physicochemical properties which are relevant to receptor binding.

Before leaving this example it is worth considering one other aspect of the analysis and that is the possibility of chance effects. The experimental data set consisted of binding results for just eight compounds* whereas the descriptor set contained 15 possible variables. Topliss and Edwards[37] have shown the danger of chance correlations using regression analysis and demonstrated the expected result that their likelihood increases as the number of screened variables increases. Since MLR is a supervised learning technique it might be reasonable to suppose that the danger of chance effects would apply to other supervised learning methods, such as PLS. Some workers have claimed that cross-validation reduces or eliminates chance effects although it is difficult to see how a technique which assesses "goodness of fit" or "robustness" can have any effect on chance probabilities. Chance effects in PLS modeling have been examined[38] and Clark and Cramer have shown that in applications of PLS to CoMFA type problems the likelihood of chance correlations decreases as the number of variables is increased.[39] This is presumably a consequence of the fact that PLS seeks to explain variance in both the x (independent) and y (dependent) data sets. Rogers has suggested (D. Rogers, personal communication.) that random shuffling of the dependent data, first suggested by Klopman,[40] is a good approach to the avoidance of chance effects. Other applications of the PLS method are discussed in the section on 3D-QSAR. But before moving on to other principal component related examples, it is worth pointing out that PLS is not restricted to the analysis of a single dependent variable. In a study of membrane toxicity Andersson and coworkers considered both the highest tolerated concentration (HTC) and the concentration which caused 20% leakage of ATP (EC_{20}) as their dependent variables.[33] They fitted a PLS model using six physicochemical descriptors (for 14 compounds) which described 71% of the combined variance of the biological data using a single latent variable.

Principal component analysis (PCA) may be used to examine the relationships between descriptor variables by inspection of a plot of the loadings of the variables on any two principal components. Figure 4.4 shows such a plot for a set of nine physicochemical descriptors used to characterize 45 carboxylic acids which had

---

* *Predictions were made for a further set of 100 possible analogues using a PLS model based on purely tabulated physicochemical properties.*

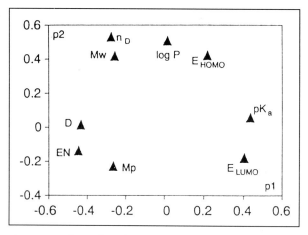

Fig. 4.4. Loadings plot of nine descriptor variables on the first two principal components. Variables are: molecular weight (Mw), melting point (Mp), density (D), refractive index (n_D), octanol/water partition coefficient (log P), acid dissociation constant (pK_a), energy of highest occupied molecular orbital (E_{HOMO}), energy of lowest unoccupied molecular orbital (E_{LUMO}) and electronegativity (EN). (Reproduced with permission from Eriksson L, Berglind R, Sjöstrom M. Chemometr & Intell Lab Syst 1994; 23:235-45. ©1994 Elsevier Science.)

the potential to cause skin corrosion.[41] The loadings plot shows some interesting groupings of variables; molecular weight and refractive index are associated together, for example, and are quite close to log P and the energy of the highest occupied molecular orbital. Density and electronegativity are correlated with one another, perhaps surprisingly, and pK_a is seen to lie quite close to the energy of the lowest unoccupied molecular orbital. A plot such as this can be very useful in showing the relationships between variables in a particular data set and the corresponding plot for the compounds (a scores plot) will similarly reveal any groupings amongst the samples. Having generated principal components they may be used as "new" variables in a number of different ways. In addition to creating scores and loadings plots, the PCs may be used in the creation of regression models (see later in this section) and as "design" variables to select compounds from the set according to some statistical experimental design. PCA on the carboxylic acid set gave three principal components which accounted for 74% of the variance in the descriptor set. Applying a 2^3 factorial design, Eriksson and coworkers selected a set of nine compounds (eight points at the vertices of the physicochemical property space plus a central point) to form a training set.[41] A smaller validation set was chosen using a half fractional factorial design (four compounds) plus an extra central point. These compounds were tested in a skin corrosion assay (rabbit) and the results analyzed using a PLS model which included nonlinear terms (see ref. 41 for details). Prediction results for the validation set, including an extra compound outside the training set domain, are shown in Table 4.2.

The data examined by PCA are not restricted to just the independent data set, or just the dependent set if there is more than one dependent variable; both types of data may be incorporated in the same analysis. Darwish and coworkers applied PCA to a set of six biological activities (inhibition after 4 and 8 days of *Aspergillus niger*, *Helminthosporium sativum* and *Bacillus subtilis*) and eight experimental (chromatographic) physicochemical properties of nine benzothiazole derivatives.[42] This gave four principal components with an eigenvalue greater than one* as shown in Table 4.3. Inspection of the table shows that the first component involves

Table 4.2. The 2^{3-1} fractional design for a validation set of carboxylic acids along with observed and predicted lowest observed effect concentrations (LOEC)

Design point	Carboxylic acid	Observed LOEC	Predicted* LOEC
– – +	Malonic	1.2	1.0
+ – –	Butyric	2.8	2.4
– + –	Dichloroacetic	1.0	1.1
+ + +	Methacrylic	2.9	2.1
0 0 0	2-Hydroxybutyric	2.4	1.6
Extra	Vinylacetic	2.9	2.9

* Predicted from a two dimensional PLS model derived from 18 chemical descriptors. (Reproduced with permission from Eriksson L, Berglind R, Sjöström M. Chemometr & Intell Lab Syst 1994; 23:235-45. ©1994 Elsevier Science.)

* *A commonly accepted criterion for "significance" but see later.*

high loadings of two of the three types of biological property and all but one of the physicochemical properties. Component two contains high loadings for the *Aspergillus niger* data as does component one, but here the signs of the loadings are reversed. The results for the two time points for *Helminthosporium sativum* both load onto the third PC and this component has little association with any of the chromatographic descriptors. The fourth component contains high loadings for two of the physicochemical properties but none of the biological results show any association with

Table 4.3. Results of the application of PCA to a combined data set of biological activities and physicochemical properties

PC No.	Eigenvalue	Variance explained (%)	Sum of explained variance
1	6.23	44.47	44.47
2	3.03	21.66	66.14
3	2.27	16.21	82.34
4	1.61	11.53	93.87

Principal component loadings*

Parameter	PC:1	2	3	4
A	**-0.57**	**0.79**	0.05	0.01
B	**-0.57**	**0.79**	0.05	0.01
C	0.13	-0.33	**0.92**	-0.07
D	0.13	-0.33	**0.92**	-0.08
E	**-0.61**	0.34	0.48	0.17
F	**-0.62**	**0.78**	0.03	0.08
G	**0.64**	0.23	0.11	**0.69**
H	0.47	0.02	-0.10	**0.79**
I	**0.73**	**0.56**	0.23	-0.28
J	**0.70**	0.47	0.05	-0.49
K	**0.78**	0.41	0.37	0.18
L	**0.94**	0.05	0.27	0.13
M	**0.93**	0.24	0.01	-0.21
N	**0.88**	0.03	-0.20	-0.22

* High loadings (above 0.5) are shown in bold.
Parameters A and B are the inhibition of *Aspergillus niger* after 4 and 8 days, C and D are 4 and 8 day results for *Helminthosporium sativum*, E and F are similarly for *Bacillus subtilis*. Parameters G to N are chromatographic parameters measured in different eluent systems.
(Reproduced with permission from Darwish Y, Cserhati T, Forgacs E. Chemometr & Intell Lab Syst 1994; 24:169-76. ©1994 Elsevier Science.)

this PC. These complex relationships between the original variables and the principal components shown in the table demonstrates one of the features of PCA, the components are merely mathematical constructs intended to explain variance in the set and they thus do not necessarily have any physical significance. Having said this, of course, it is always possible to attempt some sort of interpretation of the "meaning" of principal components and quite often it will be found that a component does represent a particular type of physicochemical property.[43]

Another way in which principal components may be used is to employ them as the independent variables in multiple linear regression analysis. Livingstone and coworkers have reported an analysis of a set of monosubstituted benzenes using computational chemistry to characterize the molecules and PCA and PLS to analyze the results.[44] Charge-transfer complex formation data (κ) were available for these compounds and this had previously been explained by three substituent constants—π, MR (a "bulk" descriptor[3]) and R (a resonance component of σ[3]):

$$\kappa = 0.04(\pm\ 0.0004)MR - 0.33(\pm\ 0.03)\pi - 0.21(\pm\ 0.06)R + 0.0 \quad (8)$$

$$n = 35 \quad r^2 = 0.95 \quad F = 76.7 \quad s = 0.1$$

PCA on the descriptor data (11 selected computed properties) gave rise to four principal components with eigenvalues greater than one and a fifth component with an eigenvalue close to one (0.95). Forward stepping regression analysis using these five PCs gave the following equations:*

$$\kappa = 0.191PC1 + 0.453 \quad\quad\quad\quad\quad\quad\quad\quad\quad\quad\quad (9)$$

$$r^2 = 0.5 \quad F = 33.0 \quad s = 0.32$$

$$\kappa = 0.191PC1 + 0.193PC4 + 0.453 \quad\quad\quad\quad\quad\quad\quad (10)$$

$$r^2 = 0.732 \quad F = 43.8 \quad s = 0.24$$

$$\kappa = 0.191PC1 + 0.193PC4 + 0.13PC5 + 0.453 \quad\quad\quad (11)$$

$$r^2 = 0.814 \quad F = 45.2 \quad s = 0.20$$

---

* *Standard errors for the regression coefficients were not reported but all* t *statistics were significant at the 1% level or better.*

There are some interesting things to note about these regression equations. The first PC contained, among other descriptors, calculated molar refractivity (CMR) which of course is equivalent to the MR term in Equation 8. The fourth PC contained a calculated log P (CLOGP) term which is equivalent to the π substituent constant in Equation 8 and thus it can be seen that the regression on principal components is giving results that are consistent with the regression analysis using "classical" substituent constant data. As regression Equations 9-11 are built up it may be seen that the regression coefficients and the constant term are unchanging. This is because the principal components are orthogonal to one another, each part of the variance in the κ values that they explain is unique to them. Finally, it should be noted that PCs two and three are not involved in these regression models. Although they are important in terms of the variance in the physicochemical descriptor set that they explain, this part of the variance is not relevant to the description of the κ data.

CLASSIFIED RESPONSE DATA

It is commonly assumed that the "Q" in QSAR refers to the biological data or at least the relationships which are generated between the response data and the physicochemical descriptors. Although this is a popular interpretation of the meaning of QSAR, it is not really true. The term quantitative refers to the use of physicochemical properties to describe changes in chemical structure (*cf.* Equation 1) and this is what distinguishes QSAR from SAR. It is therefore possible to construct QSAR models using qualitative data such as active/inactive, toxic/nontoxic, good/medium/poor, etc. or to take quantitative data and classify the compounds in the set according to some activity cut-off criteria.* It is also possible to construct QSARs without any dependent data at all! Selection of compounds for synthesis or testing on the basis of their physicochemical properties, for example. The use of classified data requires the application of different statistical methods, e.g., discriminant analysis, although a commonly seen

---

* *Some biological tests may be so variable or imprecise that it is actually an improvement to classify the data in this way.*

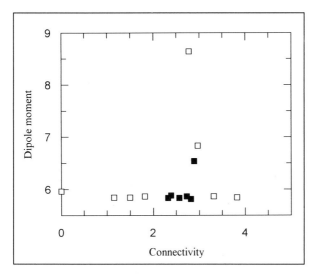

Fig. 4.5. Plot of dipole moment against the first order valence-corrected molecular connectivity index for a set of praziquantel analogues, active compounds are indicated by filled squares. (Reproduced with permission from Ordorica MA, et al. Quant Struct-Act Relat 1993; 12:246-50. ©1993 VCH).

mistake is the use of regression analysis with such data. Of course, one of the simplest ways in which classified data may be treated is to use the classification results to code the points in a plot of physicochemical descriptors. Ordorica and coworkers reported an analysis of 14 antiparasitic analogs of praziquantel which had been tested in vivo and in vitro against *Shistosoma mansoni* and *Hymenolepsis nana*.[45] Figure 4.5 shows a plot of these compounds on the best two variables selected by cluster significance analysis[46] where it can be clearly seen that the active compounds are clustered together.

Reports of the use of classified techniques are relatively rare in drug design, probably because of the misunderstanding outlined at the beginning of this section, but they are widely used in the analysis of toxicity data which is often reported as YES/NO results. The TOPKAT program from Health Designs, Inc. (Rochester, N.Y., USA) makes use of linear discriminant analysis in the mutagenicity, carcinogenicity, teratogenicity and biodegradability modules. Table 4.4 shows the results of a recent report on the predictive ability of the mutagenicity module.[47] The database consisted of 1265 compounds and the discriminant function used 91 computed features to give an average success rate of 98% (97.5% by leave-one-out cross-validation). The training set shown in Table 4.4 is smaller than the whole database because some compounds could not be characterized by the program (17) and be-

Table 4.4. Performance of the mutagenicity module of the TOPKAT program

No. of compounds in database	1265.0
No. suitable for modeling	1213.0
No. in the training set	1083.0
No. of discriminating features	91.0
Degrees of freedom	991.0
F-Ratio	61.6
Wilk's Λ-statistic	0.151

Assigned Class in training set		Predicted class in resubstitution (cross-validation)		
		Mut.	Indeterminate	Non-Mut.
Mutagenic	669	650 (648)	10 (7)	9 (14)
Non-Mutagenic	414	1 (5)	2 (1)	411 (408)

(Reproduced with permission from Enslein K, Gombar VJ, Blake BW. Mutation Res 1994; 305:47-61. ©1994 Elsevier Science.)

cause some compounds had equivocal results (35) or were found to be unduly influential on the model (130). Despite this, the remaining set of over 1000 compounds is still quite large to give such impressive prediction results. Benigni and coworkers have compared regression models for mutagenic potency with discriminant equations which predict mutagenic/non-mutagenic behavior.[29] They showed that while log P was an important determinant of potency, electronic factors such as the energy of HOMO or LUMO were more important descriptors in the discriminant functions. These findings were in general agreement with earlier work on the induction of aneuploidy in *Aspergillus nidulans*[48] and they concluded that it was necessary to consider both types of QSAR in risk assessment.

The fact that biological data sets can often be divided up into two classes which can be easily recognized in plots of two physicochemical properties (*cf*. Fig. 4.5) or 2D plots of higher dimensional spaces[49] is a great convenience to the drug designer. Unfortunately, not all data sets behave in such an obliging fashion and one of the problems with classified data is that one class may be embedded within another. This problem was addressed by Rose and coworkers who devised a technique called single class discrimination using principal components (SCD-PCA).[50] Briefly, this technique operates by centering and scaling the data set to the space occupied by the active compounds and then enhances the clustering of actives while dispersing the inactives, see reference 50 for full details. In the original report the method was applied to a set of antifilarial analogs of Antimycin A_1 for which both in vitro and in vivo data were available. Both biological responses were measured on continuous scales (EC_{50} and % worm reduction) but the data were classified into two groups by taking the top 15 and 10 most active compounds in the in vitro and in vivo sets respectively and calling these "active." Figure 4.6 shows the results of the application of this technique to the two data sets and it may be seen that the active compounds are quite tightly clustered together although some inactives are included in the active cluster for the in vitro data. These latter compounds are resolved when a third PC (3 components accounted for 94% of the variance) is used to create a 3-D plot. The problem of an embedded class can be more generally stated as the presence of two classes which are not capable of linear separation. Benigni has described a technique called EVE which is based on Euclidean distances and has applied it successfully to the same data set of praziquantel analogs shown in Figure 4.5.[51]

3D-QSAR

3D-QSAR methods have considerable appeal since although they use relatively complicated mathematical techniques, e.g., PLS in a method such as CoMFA, the results of the analysis may be presented as a picture in which regions of favorable and unfavorable interactions are shown surrounding the overlayed compounds. As a result, many reports simply present their results graphically and it is often difficult to extract the important molecular determinants of activity. Some recent papers, however, do compare the technique with "classical" QSAR treatments. Carroll and cowork-

Fig. 4.6. PC scores plot from the SCD-PCA method applied to in vitro (a) and in vivo (b) data for antifilarial activity; filled squares represent active compounds. (Reproduced with permission from Rose VS, Wood J, MacFie HJH. Quant Struct-Act Relat 1991; 10:359-68. ©1991 VCH).

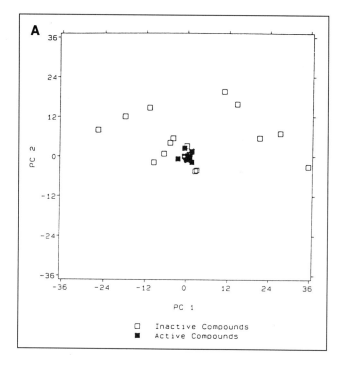

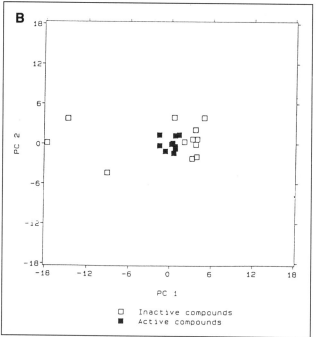

ers have studied the binding of cocaine analogs to the dopamine transport receptor in rat striatal membranes.[52] Their best multiple linear regression equation with an r^2 of 0.71 involved π and the Verloop B_4 Sterimol descriptor. A CoMFA model for the same data set gave an r^2 of 0.95 with a quite impressive plot of predicted against observed $\log(1/IC_{50})$ values over a range of ~2.5 log units. The leave-one-out cross-validated results, however, gave considerably lower r^2 values (between 0.43 and 0.57) suggesting that the CoMFA model may be overfitting the data. Agarwal and coworkers have examined the binding of tetrahydropyridinylindole derivatives to $5HT_{1A}$ and $5HT_2$ receptors and came to the conclusion that the standard Hansch approach and a CoMFA model gave comparable results.[53] Interestingly, this study made predictions of activity for new compounds using both methods and found that neither technique "appears to give noticeably better or worse predictions...based on our comparison using identical data sets." The CoMFA method has the clear advantage that it is possible to include compounds which can be overlaid with the other molecules in the set but which could not be parameterized for inclusion in a Hansch type model. The multiple regression approach using substituent constants is, in principle at least, simpler to understand and "less prone to arbitrariness in its implementation."

The selection of test and training sets is a crucial factor in the success of any QSAR technique and the CoMFA method is no exception to this. Caliendo and coworkers have examined the importance of set selection by applying the technique of factorial design to a set of 71 N-acyl-L-aminoacid esters which are hydrolyzed by the enzyme α-chymotrypsin.[54] The compounds were characterized using the CoMFA method and PCA was applied to the combined steric and electrostatic fields to produce three PCs. These PCs were used as design variables, three levels for PC1 and two levels for the other PCs, to produce a factorial design set of 12 training compounds by taking compounds which were closest (Euclidean distance) to the factorial design points. This set is referred to as set A in Table 4.5; a second set was chosen using "weighted distances" according to the eigenvalues of the PCs (set B) and 50 sets of 12 compounds were formed by random selection from the original data set of 71 compounds. Set A has a higher cross-vali-

Table 4.5. Cross-validation and prediction* results for CoMFA models derived from two factorial design training sets and selected⁺ random training sets

Set	N_{PCs}	r^2_{CV}	S_{PRED}	r^2_{PRED}
A	3	0.864	0.941	0.603
B	1	0.648	0.732	0.767
RD_5	2	0.683	1.090	0.511
RD_7	1	0.485	0.658	0.824
RD_{13}	1	0.443	1.199	0.445
RD_{22}	2	0.906	0.722	0.772
RD_{27}	2	0.776	0.615	0.837
RD_{32}	1	0.278	0.767	0.764
RD_{35}	1	0.347	1.376	0.289
RD_{40}	2	0.781	1.385	0.237
RD_{44}	2	0.615	0.564	0.869
RD_{48}	1	0.801	0.798	0.723

*N_{PCs} is the number of latent variables in the model, r^2_{CV} is the leave-one-out cross-validated correlation coefficient, S_{PRED} and r^2_{PRED} are the prediction error and correlation coefficient for prediction of the remaining "test set" of 59 compounds.
⁺Results are shown for 10 representative sets including the "best" and "worst" results.
(Adapted with permission from Caliendo G, Greco G, Novellino E et al. Quant Struct-Act Relat 1994; 13:249-61. ©1994 VCH.)

dated correlation coefficient (r^2_{CV}) than set B but a lower correlation coefficient for prediction (r^2_{PRED}) for the remaining 59 compound test set and the authors concluded that this set, which took account of the "importance" of the three PCs, was a more balanced selection. Perhaps one of the most interesting results of this study, however, is the relatively good performance of the randomly chosen training sets. Over 40% of these sets showed a comparable or superior predictive performance to set B and this was not because the sets contained common compounds. Set 44, for example, which had the highest r^2_{PRED} value had only three compounds which corresponded to those in set B. There are a number of randomly chosen sets which have a low r^2_{PRED}/r^2_{CV} ratio and this demonstrates the danger of relying on cross-validation alone to characterize how well these models fit the data.

One of the problems with 3D-QSAR techniques is the choice of probes to use in the calculation of interaction energies at the grid points surrounding the molecules. The original CoMFA method proposed the use of just steric and electrostatic probes in the perhaps not unreasonable expectation that these two types of interaction would characterize the way that a molecule would interact with some binding site. However, as shown in Table 4.1, numerous types of descriptors have been employed in successful QSAR models including in particular energies of HOMOs or LUMOs. Poso and coworkers added a LUMO field (E_{LUMO}) to the standard steric (S) and electrostatic (E) fields in a CoMFA study of mutagenic compounds.[55] The highest cross-validated r^2 was obtained for a CoMFA model containing E_{LUMO} and S fields (0.923) which compared very favorably with S (0.847) and E (0.751) fields alone and with a combined S and E model (0.791). Other factors which may affect the description of molecules using grid point energies are the spacing of the grid points and the dielectric constant term which is used in the calculation of interaction energy. Cruciani and Watson used a set of inhibitors of glycogen phosphorylase *b* for which X-ray crystal structures of the inhibitor-enzyme complex were known to investigate these factors.[56] In this study, which included an examination of variable selection procedures, it was shown that both of these factors are of importance and that the dielectric constant which produced the best prediction results was in the range 10 to 20. This reduction in dielectric from the usually chosen value of 80 which mimics bulk water presumably is a better reflection of the true dielectric nature of the binding site of the enzyme. CoMFA like approaches have also been used to try to predict more fundamental physicochemical properties, as discussed in the next section.

In addition to the CoMFA technique other methods have been employed to produce 3D-QSAR models. Good and coworkers have made use of molecular similarity measures[57] although Benigni et al demonstrated that similarity matrices neither complemented nor improved classical descriptors.[58] The hypothetical active site lattice (HASL) method has been used to predict both in vitro and in vivo results for a variety of biological activities.[59] Pharmacophore generation programs such as CATALYST from MSI, Inc. and APEX from Biosym Technologies, Inc. produce 3D-QSAR models since the molecular features identified in the training set molecules contain geometric as well as physicochemical information.[60]

PHYSICOCHEMICAL PROPERTIES

Techniques for the prediction or explanation of a complex property such as biological activity can equally well be applied to the (possibly) simpler problem of physicochemical properties. We have already seen such an example in the description of the charge-transfer substituent constant, κ, in Equations 8-11. One property that has been a particular focus for attempts at explanation and prediction, presumably because of it's importance as a descriptor of biological properties, is the partition coefficient. The techniques employed have ranged from completely empirical to theoretical and have made use of many techniques such as expert systems, PCA, multiple regression, artificial neural networks and so on. A recent study reported[32] the following regression equation:*

$$\log P = 0.01(\pm 0.0006)S - 0.001(\pm 0.0001)ES + 104(\pm 5.9)CT \quad (12)$$

$$n = 63 \quad r = 0.983 \quad s = 0.26$$

Where S and ES are terms for surface tension and electrostatic interaction calculated from electrostatic potentials and CT is a charge-transfer interaction term calculated from orbital energies and atomic areas. Since all of these terms may be calculated for any molecular structure the model shown in Equation 12 is, in principle, a "general" model for octanol/water partition coefficients and it was shown that this technique was able to calculate values for compounds which are not parameterized in the well known CLOGP technique.[61]

Another physicochemical property which has been shown to be of importance in the distribution of compounds within biological systems is the ability of particular functional groups, including ring systems, to take part in hydrogen bonding. Abraham and coworkers have published an extensive series of reports on proton donor and acceptor scales (for example, see ref. 62) and the investigation of different partition coefficient systems using the linear solvation energy relationship (LSER) approach has given insight into hydrogen bond strength and directionality.[63] The LSER

---

* *No F statistic was reported for the fit and the correlation was simply reported as the "correlation coefficient."*

technique has found many applications in the prediction and explanation of chemical properties but one drawback to this essentially empirical approach is the availability (and consistency) of experimental measurements from which the parameters are drawn. Famini and coworkers have addressed this problem by the calculation of theoretical descriptors for use in LSER type relationships (known as TLSER) and this appears to offer considerable promise.[64] The addition of a hydrogen bonding term to partition coefficient values measured in two solvent systems (ΔlogP) has been shown by different groups of workers to improve the predictive ability of models for penetration of the blood-brain barrier.[65-66]

Many other properties have been modeled ranging from soil sorption coefficients[67] to electron affinities[68] and in a recent review Dearden discusses the prediction of some quite fundamental properties such as solubility, surface tension, boiling point and so on.[69] 3D-QSAR techniques have also been used successfully in the prediction of physicochemical properties; Kim has reported[70] the modeling of partition coefficients of pyrazines and pyridines using CH_3, H^+ and H_2O probes with the program GRID (Molecular Discovery Ltd., West way house, Elms Parade, Oxford, England) and Steinmetz has used a similar system to predict the solubility and distribution characteristics of amino acids.[71]

SUMMARY

The examples shown in this chapter should give some idea of the very wide range of types of biological activity and physicochemical properties that may be modeled using regression analysis, principal component analysis and PLS, classification techniques and 3D-QSAR. In addition to this wide variety of types of biological response there is also a large range of analytical methods that may be employed in the construction of QSAR models. The examples discussed here have employed some of the more popular techniques, Table 4.6 gives a taste of some of the newer or less commonly used methods. Of course it is not possible to list every technique, just as it is impossible to list an example of every type of biological property, so if your favorite method is missing from the list it is simply because this is a somewhat arbitrary collection.

Table 4.6. Examples of some newer or less commonly used methods for the creation of QSAR models

Analytical method	Property involved	Ref.
Fuzzy Adaptive Least Squares	Anticarcinogenic arginine-vasopressin antagonists	72
Non-Linear Mapping	Compound selection	73
Structure-Activity Maps	Anti-hypertensives	74
	Sweeteners	74
Rule Induction	GABA Agonists	75
	Inotropes	75
	Antimalarials	75
MULTICASE	pK_a prediction	76
Free-Wilson	Anti-microbial	77
Neural Networks	Biodegradability	78
Evolutionary algorithm	Variable selection	79
Kohonen mapping	Hallucinogens	80
	Chemical reactivity	80
Minimal Steric Difference	Corticosteroid binding globulin	81
	Testosterone binding globulin	81
Genetic Algorithm	Antifilarial	82
	Acetylcholinesterase inhibitors	82

REFERENCES

1. Crum Brown A, Frazer T. On the connection between chemical constitution and physiological action. Part I. On the physiological action of the salts of the ammonium bases, derived from Strychnia, Brucia, Thebaia, Codeia, Morphia, and Nicotia. Trans Roy Soc Edinburgh 1868-9; 25:151-203.
2. Murugan R, Grendze MP, Toomey JE et al. Predicting physical properties from molecular structure. Chemtech 1994; June:17-23.
3. Livingstone DJ. Quantitative structure-activity relationships. In: Zalewski R, Krygowski TM, Shorter R, eds. Similarity Models in Organic Chemistry, Biochemistry and Related Fields. Amsterdam: Elsevier, 1991:557-627.
4. Kubinyi H. QSAR: Hansch Analysis and Related Approaches. Weinheim: VCH, 1993.
5. Dean P, ed. Molecular Similarity in Drug Design. London: Blackie Academic & Professional, 1995.
6. Wermuth CG, ed. Trends in QSAR and Molecular Modelling 92. Leiden: ESCOM, 1993.
7. Sanz F, ed. Trends in QSAR and Molecular Modelling 94. Barcelona: JR Prous, in press.

8. Boyd DB. Successes of computer-assisted molecular design. In: Lipkowitz KB and Boyd DB, eds. Reviews in Computational Chemistry. Weinheim: VCH, 1990: 355-71.

9. Livingstone DJ. Pattern recognition methods in rational drug design. In: Langone JJ, ed. Methods in Enzymology. Vol. 203. San Diego: Academic Press, 1991:613-38.

10. Scalzo M, Biava M, Porretta GC et al. Correlation analysis in a set of 1,5- diarylpyrroles with antimycotic activity. In: Silipo C, Vittoria A, eds. QSAR: Rational Approaches to the Design of Bioactive Compounds. Amsterdam: Elsevier, 1991:389-92.

11. Hansch C, Fujita T. ρ-σ-π Analysis. A method for the correlation of biological activity and chemical structure. J Am Chem Soc 1964; 86:1616-26.

12. Koch A, Seydel JK, Gasco A et al. QSAR and molecular modelling for a series of isomeric X-sulfanilamido-1-phenylpyrazoles. Quant Struct-Act Relat 1993; 12:373-82.

13. Livingstone DJ. The trouble with chemometrics. In: Sanz F, ed. Trends in QSAR and Molecular Modelling 94. Barcelona: JR Prous, in press.

14. Saxena AK. Physicochemical significance of topological parameters, connectivity indices and information content. Part 1: Correlation studies in the sets with aromatic and aliphatic substituents. Quant Struct-Act Relat 1995; 14:31-8.

15. Kubinyi H. The physicochemical significance of topological parameters. A rebuttal. Quant Struct-Act Relat 1995; 14:149-50.

16. De Benedetti PG, Menziani MC, Frassineti C. A quantum chemical QSAR study of carbonic anhydrase inhibition by sulfonamides. Sulfonamide carbonic anhydrase inhibitors: quantum chemical QSAR. Quant Struct-Act Relat 1985; 4:23-8.

17. Hyde RM, Livingstone DJ. Perspectives in QSAR: computer chemistry and pattern recognition. J Comp-Aided Mol Design 1988; 2:145-55.

18. Kikuchi O. Systematic QSAR procedures with quantum chemical descriptors. Quant Struct-Act Relat 1987; 6:179-84.

19. Ford MG, Livingstone DJ. Multivariate techniques for parameter selection and data analysis exemplified by a study of pyrethroid neurotoxicity. Quant Struct-Act Relat 1990; 9:107-14.

20. Cocchi M, Menziani MC, De Benedetti PG et al. Theoretical versus empirical molecular descriptors in monosubstituted benzenes. A chemometric study. Chemometr & Intell Lab Syst 1992; 14:209-24.

21. Barratt MD. A quantitative structure-activity relationship (QSAR) for prediction of α-2μ-globulin nephropathy. Quant Struct-Act Relat 1994; 13:275-80.

22. De Benedetti PG, Cocchi M, Menziani MC et al. Theoretical quantitative size and shape activity and selectivity analyses of 5-HT1A serotonin and α1-adrenergic receptor ligands. J Mol Struct (Theochem) 1994; 305:101-10.

23. Hopfinger AJ, Kawakami Y. QSAR analysis of a set of benzothiopyranoindazole anti-cancer analogs based upon their DNA intercalation properties as determined by molecular dynamics simulation. Anti-Cancer Drug Des 1992; 7:203-17.

24. Hudson BD, George AR, Ford MG et al. Structure-activity relationships of pyrethroid insecticides. Part 2. The use of molecular dynamics for conformation searching and average parameter calculation. J Comp-aided Mol Design 1992; 6:191-201.

25. Yoneda F, Nitta Y. Electronic structure and antibacterial activity of nitrofuran derivatives. Chem Pharm Bull 1964; 12:1264-8.

26. Joshi RK, Meister T, Scapozza L et al. A new quantum chemical approach in QSAR-analysis. Parameterisation of conformational energies into molecular descriptors Jmn (steric) and Jsn (electronic). Arzneim Forsch 1994; 44:779-90.

27. Seri-Levy A, West S, Richards WG. Molecular similarity, quantitative chirality, and QSAR for chiral drugs. J Med Chem 1994; 37:1727-32.

28. Hansch C, Telzer BR, Zhang L. Comparative QSAR in toxicology: Examples from teratology and cancer chemotherapy of aniline mustards. Crit Rev Toxicol 1995; 25:67-89.

29. Benigni R, Andreoli C, Giuliani A. QSAR models for both mutagenic potency and activity: application to nitroarenes and aromatic amines. Environ Mol Mutagen 1994; 24:208-19.

30. Feriani A, Gaviraghi G. Lacidipine, a long-acting 1,4-dihydropyridine calcium antagonist: structure-activity studies. La Chimica & L'Industria 1993; 75:393-7.

31. Hopfinger AJ, Burke BJ, Dunn WJ. A generalized formalism of three-dimensional quantitative structure-property relationship analysis for flexible molecules using tensor representation. J Med Chem 1994; 37:3768-74.

32. Sasaki Y, Kubodera H, Matuszaki T et al. Prediction of octanol/water partition coefficients using parameters derived from molecular structures. J Pharmacobio-Dyn 1991; 14:207-14.

33. Andersson M, Bocchio F, Sterner O et al. Structure-activity relationships for unsaturated dialdehydes 7. The membrane toxicity of 15 sesquiterpenoids measured as the induction of ATP leakage in ELD cells. The correlation of the activity with structural descriptors by the multivariate PLS method. Toxic in Vitro 1993; 7:1-6.

34. A-Razzak M, Glen RC. Applications of rule-induction in the derivation of quantitative structure-activity relationships. J Comp-Aided Mol Design 1992; 6:349-83.

35. Hansch C, Klein TE. Quantitative structure-activity relationships and molecular graphics in evaluation of enzyme-ligand interactions. In: Langone JJ, ed. Methods in Enzymology. Vol. 202. San Diego: Academic Press, 1991:512-43.

36. Bordi F, Mor M, Morini G et al. QSAR study on H3-receptor affinity of benzothiazole derivatives of thioperamide. Il Farmaco 1994; 49:153-66.

37. Topliss JG, Edwards RP. Chance factors in studies of quantitative structure-activity relationships. J Med Chem 1979; 22:1238-44.

38. Wakeling IN, Morris JJ. A test of significance for partial least squares regression. J Chemometr 1993; 7:291-304.

39. Clark M, Cramer RD. The probability of chance correlation using partial least squares. Quant Struct-Act Relat 1993; 12:137-45.

40. Klopman G, Kalos AN. Causality in structure-activity studies. J Comp Chem 1985; 6:492-506.

41. Eriksson L, Berglind R, Sjöstrom M. A multivariate quantitative structure-activity relationship for corrosive carboxylic acids. Chemometr & Intell Lab Syst 1994; 23:235-45.

42. Darwish Y, Cserhati T, Forgacs E. Use of principal component analysis and cluster analysis in quantitative structure activity relationships: a comparative study. Chemometr & Intell Lab Syst 1994; 24:169-76.

43. van de Waterbeemd H, El Tayar N, Carrupt P-A et al. Pattern recognition study of QSAR substituent descriptors. J Comp-Aided Mol Design 1989; 3:111-32.

44. Livingstone DJ, Evans DA, Saunders MR. Investigation of a charge-transfer substituent constant using computational chemistry and pattern recognition techniques. J Chem Soc Perkin Trans 2 1992; 1545-50.

45. Ordorica MA, Velasquez ML, Ordorica JG et al. A principal component and cluster significance analysis of the antiparasitic potency of praziquantel and some analogs. Quant Struct-Act Relat 1993; 12:246-50.

46. McFarland JW, Gans DJ. Cluster significance analysis: a new QSAR tool for asymmetric data sets. Drug Inf J 1990; 24:705-11.

47. Enslein K, Gombar VJ, Blake BW. Use of SAR in computer-assisted prediction of carcinogenicity and mutagenicity of chemicals by the TOPKAT program. Mutation Res 1994; 305:47-61.

48. Benigni R, Andreoli C, Conti L et al. Quantitative structure-activity relationship models corrrectly predict the toxic and aneuploidizing properties of six halogenated methanes in *Aspergillus nidulans*. Mutagenesis 1993; 8:301-5.

49. Hudson B, Livingstone DJ, Rahr E. Pattern recognition display methods for the analysis of computed molecular properties. J Comp-Aided Mol Design 1989; 3:55-65.

50. Rose VS, Wood J, MacFie HJH. Single class discrimination using principal component analysis (SCD-PCA). Quant Struct-Act Relat 1991; 10:359-68.

51. Benigni R. EVE, a distance based approach for discriminating nonlinearly separable groups. Quant Struct-Act Relat 1994; 13:406-11.

52. Carroll FI, Gao Y, Rahman MA et al. Synthesis, ligand binding, QSAR, and CoMFA study of 3β-(*p*-substituted phenyl)tropane-2β-carboxylic acid methyl esters. J Med Chem 1991; 34:2719-25.

53. Agarwal A, Pearson PP, Taylor EW et al. Three-dimensional quantitative structure-activity relationships of 5-HT receptor binding data for tetrahydropyridinylindole derivatives: a comparison of the Hansch and CoMFA methods. J Med Chem 1993; 36:4006-14.

54. Caliendo G, Greco G, Novellino E et al. Combined use of factorial design and comparative molecular field analysis (CoMFA): a case study. Quant Struct-Act Relat 1994; 13:249-61.

55. Poso A, Tuppurainen K, Gynther J. Modelling of molecular mutagenicity with comparative molecular field analysis (CoMFA). Structural and electronic properties of MX compounds related to TA100 mutagenicity. J Mol Struct (Theochem) 1994; 304:255-60.

56. Cruciani G, Watson KA. Comparative molecular field analysis using GRID force-field and GOLPE variable selection methods in a study of glycogen phosphorylase *b*. J Med Chem 1994; 37:2589-2601.

57. Good AC, Peterson SJ, Richards WG. QSAR's from molecular similarity matrices. Technique and application in the comparison of different similarity evaluation methods. J Med Chem 1993; 36:2929-37.

58. Benigni R, Cotta-Ramusino M, Giorgi F at al. Molecular similarity matrices and quantitative structure-activity relationships: a case study with methodological implications. J Med Chem 1995; 38:629-35.

59. Doweyko AM. The hypothetical active site lattice—in vitro and in vivo explorations using a three-dimensional QSAR technique. J Math Chem 1991; 7:273-85.

60. Livingstone DJ. Computational techniques for the prediction of toxicity. Toxic in Vitro 1994; 8:873-7.

61. Leo AJ. Computer calculation of peptide hydrophobicity. In: Silipo C, Vittoria A, eds. QSAR: Rational Approaches to the Design of Bioactive Compounds. Amsterdam: Elsevier, 1991:349-52.

62. Abraham MH, Duce PP, Prior DV et al. Hydrogen bonding. Part 9. Solute proton donor and proton acceptor scales for use in drug design. J Chem Soc Perkin Trans 2 1989:1355-75.

63. Leahy DE, Morris JJ, Taylor PJ et al. Model solvent systems for QSAR. Part 3. An LSER analysis of the "critical quartet." New

light on hydrogen bond strength and directionality. J Chem Soc Perkin Trans 2 1992:705-22.

64. Famini GR, Penski, CA, Wilson LY. Using theoretical descriptors in quantitative structure activity relationships: some physicochemical properties. J Phys Org Chem 1992; 5:395-408.

65. van de Waterbeemd H, Kansy M. Hydrogen-bonding capacity and brain penetration. Chimia 1992; 46:299-303.

66. Abraham MH, Chadha HS, Mitchell RC. Hydrogen bonding: 33 factors that influence the distribution of solutes between blood and brain. J Pharm Sci 1994; 83:1257-68.

67. Reddy KN, Locke MA. Prediction of soil sorption (KOC) of herbicides using semiempirical molecular properties. Weed Sci 1994; 42:453-61.

68. Hilal SH, Carreira LA, Karickhoff SW et al. Estimation of electron affinity based on structure activity relationships. Quant Struct-Act Relat 1993; 12:389-96.

69. Dearden JC. Applications of quantitative structure-property relationships to pharmaceutics. Chemometr & Intell Lab Syst 1994; 24:77-87.

70. Kim KH. Description of the reversed-phase high-performance liquid chromatography (RP-HPLC) capacity factors and octanol-water partition coefficients of 2-pyrazine and 2-pyridine analogs directly from the three-dimensional structures using comparative molecular field analysis (CoMFA) approach. Quant Struct-Act Relat 1995; 14:8-18.

71. Steinmetz WE. A CoMFA analysis of selected physical properties of amino acids in water. Quant Struct-Act Relat 1995; 14:19-23.

72. Moriguchi I, Hirono S, Liu Q et al. Fuzzy adaptive least squares and its use in quantitative structure-activity relationships. Chem Pharm Bull 1990; 38:3373-9.

73. Domine D, Devillers J, Chastrette M. A nonlinear map of substituent constants for selecting test series and deriving structure-activity relationships. 1 Aromatic series. J Med Chem 1994; 37:973-80.

74. Johnson M. Structure-activity maps for visualizing the graph variables arising in drug design. J Biopharm Stat 1993; 3:203-36.

75. A-Razzak M, Glen RC. Applications of rule-induction in the derivation of quantitative structure-activity relationships. J Comp-Aided Mol Design 1992; 6:349-83.

76. Klopman G. MULTICASE 1. A hierarchical computer automated structure evaluation program. Quant Struct-Act Relat 1992; 11:176-184.

77. Rozenski J, de Ranter CJ, Verplanken H. Quantitative structure-activity relationships for antimicrobial nitroheterocyclic drugs. Quant Struct-Act Relat 1995; 14:134-41.

78. Cambon B, Devillers J. New trends in structure-biodegradability relationships. Quant Struct-Act Relat 1993; 12:49-56.
79. Kubinyi H. Variable selection in QSAR studies. II. A highly efficient combination of systematic search and evolution. Quant Struct-Act Relat 1994; 13:393-401.
80. Bienfait B. Applications of high resolution self-organizing maps to retrosynthetic and QSAR analysis. J Chem Inf Comput Sci 1994; 34:890-98.
81. Oprea TI, Ciubotariu D, Sulea TI et al. Comparison of the minimal steric difference (MTD) and comparative molecular field analysis (CoMFA) methods for analysis of binding of steroids to carrier proteins. Quant Struct-Act Relat 1993; 12:21-6.
82. Rogers D, Hopfinger AJ. Application of genetic function approximation to quantitative structure-activity relationships and quantitative structure-property relationships. J Chem Inf Comput Sci 1994; 34:854-56.

CHAPTER 5

Recent Developments in 3D-QSAR

C. John Blankley

BACKGROUND

INTRODUCTION

The seminal papers of Hansch and Fujita,[1] Free and Wilson[2] in 1964 marked the first successful general application of theoretical and computational methods to understanding and predicting drug activity and ushered in the era of quantitative structure activity relationships (QSAR). QSAR methods have found broad applicability and success not only in the field of medicinal chemistry, but also in agricultural, toxicological and ecological areas.[3-5] The ability to relate changes in biological effect to changes in structure by consistent physicochemical models as had been achieved earlier for chemical reactivity in physical organic chemistry had eluded all earlier attempts. The insights of Hansch and Fujita into the importance of lipophilicity in drug action gleaned from earlier reported studies and the formulation of a multiple linear regression (MLR) model including hydrophobic, electronic and steric factors provided the key to uncovering such relationships. The demonstration over the subsequent years of the broad applicability of this model has made these methods a standard part of medicinal chemistry practice.

Structure-Property Correlations in Drug Research, edited by Han van de Waterbeemd. © 1996 R.G. Landes Company.

From the beginning, however, it was well recognized that the Hansch equation was only a rough first approximation to correlating biological effects with structure or properties, and among the "awkward" effects to parameterize were the steric factors, due primarily to their local and directional nature (see for example Blaney and Hansch: "Steric interactions between ligand and receptor have always been the ominous dark cloud hanging over QSAR" ref. 6, pg. 493). Also, it was recognized that the most convenient electronic parameterization, namely the substituent effect parameters derived by the Hammett relationship for substituents on aromatic rings and the Taft equations for groups in aliphatic systems, might have questionable relevance in cases where inter- rather than intramolecular interactions were involved. Furthermore, there were no convenient parameters for such important effects as hydrogen bonding, shape and the like, to say nothing about dealing with molecular flexibility, all of which are known to be important determinants of molecular recognition and interaction. Hence, it is not surprising in retrospect that, as experience developed, it turned out that the Hansch relationship was more reliably successful where lipophilicity (a whole molecule property) was the dominating effect, or in enzymatic reactivity correlations where the electronic effects of substituents have a sensible parallel to the methods used to derive them by influencing chemical reactivity at a reaction center. Much more challenging has been the derivation of convincing Hansch relationships with such important classes of biological activity as receptor binding or intrinsic activity at receptors where it is well appreciated that specific intermolecular recognition factors and interactions (steric and electronic) provide the bulk of the binding energy, and the three-dimensional (3D) shape of the ligand is critical. Even so, the Hansch equation continues to be applied fruitfully to such data and the QSAR database compiled by the Pomona group and available through BioByte Corp. catalogs over 3,000 published biological QSAR studies[7] (see also ref. 5).

The Free-Wilson approach differs from the Hansch approach in associating activity variations directly with structure, as opposed to properties. The rather more limited molecular description, and inability to extrapolate a successful result beyond the space of the

originally included substituents or groups has made this a much
less preferred and utilized method, in spite of its lack of requirement for independently determined molecular parameters. The
general linear model used, however, although it is more restrictive
in providing a flexible account of nonlinearities which frequently
intervene in biological correlations, is also more general in that it
encompasses the linear Hansch model as a special case and provides a means to incorporate additional poorly understood effects.
A good review of this method is provided by Kubinyi.[3,8] The key
element, explicit in the Free-Wilson method, but only implicit in
the Hansch method is the necessity of mapping the series of molecules to a common template. If local properties or interactions
are responsible for the biological activity variations of a set of
molecules, it is critical that the molecular regions in each molecule participating in the particular interaction be properly matched.
For homologous series, there is usually a molecular scaffold in
common which can be used as the reference, but even here, elements of symmetry can lead to alternative choices, and if the structural changes on the scaffold become large, it becomes more risky
to assume that the apparent superposition will be maintained. As
much as anything else, failure to obtain significant QSARs or, in
the more fortunate case, the observations of outliers to a QSAR
equation, can be traced to such situations. These problems can
frequently be masked by the common practice of incorporating
indicator variables which account for a systematic deviation due
to a structural feature. It is uncommon however that true parallel-
ism between the subsets thus created in the regression is verified.

   Almost from the beginning, attempts were made to incorporate the 3D component into QSAR models. Earliest, of course,
were attempts to identify steric parameters from the tradition of
physical organic chemistry. Molar refractivity was proposed as a
size parameter by Hansch, as was Taft's E_s, derived from the steric
retardation of esterification or hydrolysis of acetic acids The introduction of STERIMOL parameters by Verloop[9] provided the first
general proposal for a calculable, geometric parameter for substituents. Much work on modeling steric effects was stimulated by this
need, and Charton developed his extensive contribution to the

analysis and extension of the Taft work with his υ parameter which combines both experimental and computational elements. This was later supplemented by a plethora of branching parameters for "finer tuning" of steric effects.[10] The evolution of these and other approaches is summarized by Silipo and Vittoria.[11] Although the proposal of novel steric parameters continues today.[12-14] The search for "true" 3D-QSAR has taken several entirely new directions.

It is interesting that, at the time of publication of the six-volume set of *Comprehensive Medicinal Chemistry*, edited by Hansch, Sammes and Taylor,[15] and especially Volume 4 dealing with quantitative drug design, no mention was made of the methods we now associate most closely with 3D-QSAR. Within just three years after the publication of this work, these more ambitious approaches to incorporating the 3D nature of molecules into a correlation framework have already received a comprehensive major review edited by Kubinyi,[16] attesting to the explosion of interest in the development of these techniques. The Kubinyi volume should be required reading for all who would practice 3D-QSAR since it covers not only the specific methods in use, but also a variety of important related topics whose understanding is of critical importance in performing such analyses and interpreting their results. The field has continued to produce new developments at a rapid pace. This review will concentrate primarily on developments in the area which postdate the discussions in this review.

Certainly, the dominant 3D-QSAR method in use currently is Comparative Field Analysis (CoMFA), developed by Cramer and his associates.[17,18] This method is available commercially as an integrated part of a suite of molecular modeling programs in widespread use,[19] and because of this as well as its conceptual attractiveness it has been more widely applied than any other method. The background and origin of this method is described by Cramer[20] in the Kubinyi volume cited above. A large portion of this review will cover reports on experience with CoMFA and closely related variants with particular emphasis on attempts to come to grips with the issues and problems which are well recognized to accompany its use. CoMFA, however, is by no means the only approach to 3D-QSAR, and an update on results from and proposals for alternate methodologies will also be provided.

FORERUNNERS

The rise of molecular modeling in conjunction with the development of sophisticated and affordable computer graphics capabilities allowed for the explicit study of the geometric aspects of molecular comparison and interaction, and such methods have rapidly become established as standard tools for medicinal chemistry.[21,22] In these methods, molecules are studied by conformational analysis, superposition and docking procedures, and relative energies are used as criteria for validity. The correlations between structure and activity, however, are generally qualitative in nature, with differences in activity between analogs being attributed to differences in shape or pattern. Hansch and his group early recognized the utility of such modeling in interpreting the meaning of the physicochemical terms of a QSAR correlation, and they subsequently examined many QSARs when detailed crystallographic data became available. Favorable and unfavorable QSAR terms were interpreted in reference to experimental 3D structures with ligands modeled in, and used to refine the QSAR models themselves.[6,23] The tools to bring these two disciplines together explicitly and quantitatively, however, were lacking.

Of the attempts preceding the development of CoMFA that sought to find an explicit 3D framework for QSAR studies, three stand out as particularly significant and at least partially successful. These are the minimal topological distance (MTD) and related hyperstructure methods introduced by Simon and his colleagues,[24] molecular shape analysis (MSA) devised by Hopfinger et al[25] and the distance geometry method developed by Crippen et al.[26,27] The basis and development of each of these is covered in cited chapters of the Kubinyi volume. Each has continued to evolve in the hands of the originators.

The MTD method maps a series of related structures onto their maximal common structural graph to generate a hyperstructure representing a topological union of all analogs. Non-common nodes (generally atoms) are assigned one of three Free-Wilson-like occupancy values. These are interpreted as cavity vertices (-1), wall vertices (+1) and exterior (solvent exposed) vertices (0). The MTD for a given molecule combines the total number of cavity vertices with the sum of the node values and is purely a measure of the steric difference (misfit) from the hyperstructure. The optimal assignment of node values to the hyperstructure is obtained by an iterative process which maximizes correlation with activity. No account is made of atom type or property at a particular node. Once determined, the MTD is incorporated as a steric parameter in a standard Hansch equation, where appropriate parameters for other effects may be included. The mapping procedure, based as it is on the structural graph, pretty much limits this method to recognizably homologous series, and works best when there is only a low degree of flexibility in the set of structures. Since nodes are derived by superimposing atomic positions, approximations and ambiguities are bound to arise when flexible side chains or different sized rings must be matched. This increases the alignment possibilities that must be examined and increases the opportunity for chance correlations in the Topliss and Edwards sense.[28,29] A cross-validation procedure has been implemented in recent applications of this method to guard against this possibility. Recent applications of this method have appeared,[30,31] including one which compares MTD to CoMFA.[32] Similar numerical performance was obtained by both methods, but interpretive conclusions differed.

Molecular shape analysis (MSA) was introduced by Hopfinger and coworkers[25,33] and uses conformational analysis of a set of ligands, coupled with pairwise comparison to a reference molecule to generate a shape similarity measure. This is then used in a standard MLR equation with or without additional property variables. Iterative derivation of the equation using different shape reference molecules seeks to derive a unique conformer for each molecule which best correlates with activity. New applications of this method have been reported.[34-36] Hopfinger has recently proposed an ambitious comprehensive theoretical framework for QSAR as the latest development of his approach to this subject.[37]

Crippen adopted a different perspective in introducing distance geometry to the derivation of QSARs in the early 1980s.[27] This method focuses on binding sites of receptors and binding modes of ligands in contrast to the direct comparisons of ligand similarity which are the basis of most other approaches. The aim is to derive a sufficient number of site points around a set of ligands such that the binding energy of interaction could be derived from

the sum of interaction energies of the molecule with the site points. Each site point has a characteristic balance of physicochemically derived interaction properties, typically terms for lipophilicity (log P), steric/size (MR) and electrostatic interactions (atomic partial charge), and corresponds to a binding region on the unknown receptor. Multiple conformations of a flexible ligand are considered. The embedding routines of distance geometry are used to match the site pockets for hypothesized binding modes within a chosen distance tolerance, and then the interaction energies, including terms for both conformational energy and atomic interaction, are optimized to select the best among the binding possibilities available to a given molecule. Thus, this method provides an unbiased way both to identify a pharmacophore and to quantitatively estimate ligand potency. A variation on this approach has been elaborated by Ghose and Crippen[38] under the name of REMOTEDISC, which introduces some practical restraints to enable solutions to be more easily achieved. Ghose et al has reported applications of this method.[39-41] One other group has reported successful applications of a modified version of Crippen's method to the analysis of β-adrenergic receptor ligands.[42,43]

Crippen has moved beyond the distance geometry approach to a closer examination of the notion of minimal binding site models which has resulted in the development of the technique of Voronoi binding site modeling.[44,45] This method is particularly concerned with the problem of alternate and/or optimal binding modes for sets of compounds, and unbiased ways to deduce them.[45] Unlike most 3D methods, the alignment criterion is mathematical in nature, and only deals with subregions of the structures included. It is a very computationally-intensive method. Several recent applications have been published,[27,46-48] including an analysis of cocaine analogs binding to the dopamine transporter previously subjected to a CoMFA analysis.[46,49] The latter paper proposes a novel method for choosing robust and predictive models when several alternatives are feasible. It also illustrates the different perspective of the Voronoi approach to 3D-QSAR. The most recent evolution of Crippen's thinking is contained in yet a further development along the same lines.[50] This method, based on intervals of internal distances, concentrates on determining in an unbiased way all

feasible site models and binding modes for a given set of data which
are consistent with the quality of the data, and is illustrated on
the same data set of cocaine analogs studied by the Voronoi technique. Crippen's work, though highly mathematical in concept is
important in that it takes a unique perspective in wrestling with
some of the more vexing conceptual issues and assumptions which
underlie the enterprise of comparing molecules and binding modes.

NEWER 3D-QSAR METHODS

GENERAL CONSIDERATIONS

Ever since the arrival of molecular modeling on the medicinal
chemistry scene, there has been the desire to marry the quantitative aspects of QSAR to shape-based pharmacophores. Of the
methods mentioned above, only the distance geometry approach
explicitly incorporated both features in the same method. The
method, while unbiased, is mathematically and computationally
complex, and still depends on approximate empirical methods to
estimate binding energies. Also, the undetermined, often large
number of site-points required to adequately describe the molecules in a data set is, even today, difficult to deal with, both inter-
pretively and computationally. To some degree this has improved
in the later variants of this method, usually at the expense of re-
stricting the possible solutions. In spite of its conceptual and theoretical attractiveness, this method has not found wide use, however. The current resurgence of research into 3D-QSAR methods
stems from a shift in perspective on how to approach such a problem from an atom and group basis for comparison and matching
to a molecular field basis. This derives from the reasonable hypothesis that molecules recognize each other by virtue of the
complementarity of the energetic fields which surround them. Fields
represent a continuum of values for a particular property projected
beyond the molecular boundaries from the atoms or fragments
which constitute the molecule. Values are obtained by projecting
atom or bond-centered properties, modulated by a distance function, outside of the molecule, and summing over all atoms (bonds).
Common examples are electric fields and electrostatic potential,
which are available from quantum mechanical calculations. The

development of mathematical methods to analyze and characterize such fields in a manner suitable for incorporation into the QSAR formalism originated by Hansch has provided the key to the success of the new approaches. Fields can also be generated by using a probe with specified properties to assess an interaction energy with a property field at any point in space. A regular grid lattice is the most common framework for sampling field values. The values so obtained can be used for computation or for display on a computer graphics terminal by contouring isovalued regions. Some useful general discussions on the generation and properties of molecular fields of relevance to 3D-QSAR are available.[51-55]

CoMFA

The precursor to the most popular method of 3D-QSAR in use today, Comparative Field Analysis, was reported by Cramer as the DYLLOMS method.[17,20] This was based on the concept alluded to above of surrounding a set of molecules, aligned by some consistent rule, with a cubic lattice of points and then calculating at each of these points for each molecule an energy of interaction with an external probe molecule. Primary intermolecular interactions were postulated to be of two types; steric, as represented by the van der Waals interaction with a spherical probe, and electrostatic, as approximated by the interaction with a unit electric charge. A single probe the size of a methyl group and bearing a unit positive charge is implemented currently in Sybyl for this purpose. Grid points with high variation are then identified and these are treated as parameters in a MLR equation to search for points or regions which correlate with activity. This original approach, though attractive in principle, foundered on the volume of data, and concerns about the over-determination of the problem and chance correlation probabilities. This method was revised and made operational only when the partial least squares (PLS) method of Wold and his group[56] became available to ease the statistical concerns and advances in computer capability and molecular modeling methodology made such computationally intensive methods practical. Thus was the CoMFA method born.[18,20] In the following, recent developments in CoMFA methodology and applications will be surveyed. Those reports not covered by the review of CoMFA applications by Thibaut[57] in the Kubinyi review will be the primary focus.

CoMFA Methodology

The key steps in performing a CoMFA analysis are:

1. Choose a training set of molecules and obtain a 3D structure of each (this may also include molecules to be tested or predicted by the model).

2. Derive atomic partial charges so that an electrostatic field may be generated. (Fields of other types may also be used and examples of these are cited below.)

3. Perform conformational analysis for flexible molecules to identify for each low energy conformers as candidates for comparison.

4. Establish a consistent alignment rule(s) for all of the molecules in the set. Alignments may be derived from many sources (atom or functional group superposition, pharmacophore map, optimum field concordance, experimental nmr or X-ray structure in a bound state).

5. Select a region of interest or relevance surrounding the union volume of the analysis set and superimpose a cubic lattice of points at which to sample field values.

6. Generate the field values using a probe with relevant properties. The program default is a pseudo methyl group with a unit positive charge which determines both a steric interaction energy based on a Lennard-Jones potential and an electrostatic interaction energy based on a coulombic potential.

7. Do a statistical analysis of the resulting set of grid point interaction energies by the PLS method and examine the results. The usual techniques for evaluating standard MLR or PLS analyses may then be employed, including statistics for goodness of fit, examination of residuals and/or outliers, etc.

8. Display results as contour plots in the lattice space viewed in juxtaposition with individual molecules in the series. Regions of positive and negative steric and electrostatic contribution are thus visualized in relation to

the structures. Several options for display exist, including using actual field values or contribution to the correlation function.[20]

9. Predict additional molecules not included in the derivation of the model by suitable alignment with the training set and processing through the same sequence of transformations. Such predictions provide a means not only for estimating activities of new analogs of interest, but also for validating the true predictive capability of the model. Accurate predictions can only be expected for molecules occupying the same region as the training set.

A CoMFA analysis in its standard implementation is typically run by setting up an initial alignment of the chosen training set with its defined region, fields and program options, and then running a cross-validated analysis to determine whether an acceptable (> 0.3) cross-validated R^2 (R^2_{cv} or Q^2) can be obtained, and if so, the optimal number of components for the model. This is usually taken to be that number where Q^2 or s_{cv} (cross-validated standard error) is a maximum or minimum, respectively, or, if there is no optimum, the number where no significant improvement, (< 5% has been suggested), is observed. At this point, depending on the result, examination of residuals for a cross-validated run with the optimal number of components may suggest ways to refine or improve the model. This is most often accomplished either by identifying and removing or realigning strong outliers or examining a different alignment rule. When an acceptable Q^2 is obtained and the number of components is determined, the analysis is rerun without cross-validation using the optimum number of components to determine the standard regression statistics. The bootstrapping technique is employed to obtain estimates for the standard errors of both the coefficients and the statistics. Results are visualized graphically by displaying them as 3D-contour maps of various sorts superimposed on analogs of interest to highlight the sign and magnitude of the individual field value contributions to activity. Details and variations are surveyed by Cramer[20] and in the documentation to the program.[19]

Alternate implementations of the CoMFA technique besides the original version embodied commercially in the Tripos QSAR module appear in the literature under the CoMFA heading. It is important to understand the variations in approach in order to compare results. For example, the substantial body of work on CoMFA reported from the Abbott group uses an in-house implementation employing Goodford's GRID[58-61] fields often referred to as GRID/CoMFA and reports results in the form of principal property-like equations in the latent variables (see, for example ref. 62, and below). Field weighting issues are circumvented since the GRID fields are all calculated on a common energy scale. Norinder similarly uses his own implementation of the method, also reporting results in the latent variable mode,[63] as does a group at Fisons.[64,65] These contrast with the Tripos implementation which does all of the latent variable extraction in the background, and then reports the composite results in total field contributions for all components chosen. It is possible to examine the latent variables numerically, but analysis of their composition is not straightforward or common in reported studies using standard CoMFA. Yet another variant has been incorporated in the program PRO_LIGAND.[66]

CoMFA Fields

As originally formulated, the CoMFA method assumed that all significant intermolecular interactions could be subsumed into a steric fit (van der Waals) term and an electrostatic attraction/repulsion term. It is interesting to survey in the published examples how well this assumption has held up. Surprisingly, the bulk of analyses, especially ones that do not venture far beyond the default options provided by the program, seem to show that most "significant" results are weighted highly in favor of the steric term, or at best give a roughly equal contribution from both terms. It is rare that a significant contribution of the electronic term is found, even with appropriate scaling of the two fields. It is important to note that the electrostatic field will be sensitive to the atom charges used or the method used to calculate them. There is great variation in the published literature concerning the charge source chosen. These range from very simple charges such as those derived from the Gasteiger/Marsili procedure[67] through semi-empirical methods like MNDO or AM1 to ab initio level, with the former being the most common. It seems likely that the relatively poor performance of the electrostatic fields in reported CoMFAs may be due in part to the quality of the charge representation. Although some studies have examined more than one charge calculation method, surprisingly, it is not always found that better quality charges give better results.

Other fields have been proposed for use in CoMFA. For example, it has been found now that the original assumption that all important interactions could be contained in the combination of steric and electrostatic fields is not generally true, and that, in particular, hydrophobicity is imperfectly represented. The alternatives fields with the most published information are the GRIN/GRID fields of Goodford and the HINT hydrophobic field of Kellogg and Abraham.[53,68,69] GRID probes have been empirically parameterized to mimic specific functional group interactions found in protein structures. These probes generate interaction fields similar to those generated by SYBYL. GRID fields have been preferred in the modified CoMFA analyses from one laboratory (Kim, Martin et al), but have also been used by other groups[64,70-72] The probes chosen parallel the standard CoMFA probes (CH_3 for steric, H^+ for electrostatic) with the addition of an H_2O probe to represent a hydrogen bonding field. The three fields are separately generated. The GRID fields have proved to perform better than the standard CoMFA fields when hydrophobic interactions are important; the results of one head-to-head comparison illustrate this.[73] For steric and electrostatic effects, similar results are obtained from the two field types. A limitation of the current implementation of CoMFA is that only two fields are allowed for in the processing of the data matrix. This hinders attempts to mix fields from different sources. Other CoMFA implementations can do this easily. It has been claimed that GRID fields provide a more tailored approach to defining intermolecular interactions and are more suitable for differentiating hydrophobic or H-bonding effects which are not explicitly a part of standard CoMFA, particularly since they have been demonstrated to give good QSARs where lipophilicity is known to be the dominating effect. The current release of the GRIN/GRID programs[74] contains an interface to the SYBYL 3D-QSAR (CoMFA) module.

A direct characterization of hydrophobicity in terms of molecular fields is HINT[69] whose fields are derived from atom contributions to hydrophobicity. The latter were derived from an analysis of octanol/water partition coefficients, and provide another alternative for incorporating hydrophobic interactions explicitly. The latest version of this program also contains a CoMFA interface.[75] Several instances have now been reported where hydrophobic fields have given improved correlations over standard CoMFA fields, or if used in conjunction with these, have been the dominant contributor. An alternate hydrophobic field, the molecular lipophilicity potential (MLP) has also been introduced for use in CoMFA studies.[76]

An interesting study bears on the use of fields to calculate H-bonding ability of heterocycles.[77] In examining the ability of calculated electrostatic potentials to reproduce experimental H-bond basicity of nitrogen heterocycles, it was found that the electrostatic minima which best correlated with the experimental data were located within the van der Waals envelop of nitrogen. CoMFA ignores electrostatic contributions within the van der Waals radius of a molecule. If the typical grid spacing of 2Å and cutoff of electrostatic field at the van der Waals surface is used as is common in CoMFA, these significant electrostatic contributions may be totally missed.

HOMO fields were examined by Waller and Marshall for their utility in improving the CoMFA models of ACE inhibitors and thermolysin inhibitors.[78] This field, in conjunction with a desolvation energy term calculated by DELPHI, gave an improved predictive model for a structurally diverse set of ACE inhibitors. The HOMO field did not similarly improve the CoMFA for thermolysin inhibitors. A LUMO field was examined with less success by Poso.[79]

Alignment Rules

As noted above, CoMFA may be viewed as an attempt to marry the disciplines of QSAR and molecular modeling. The techniques of molecular superposition to derive pharmacophores have developed in parallel to QSAR and are now also standard practice in medicinal chemistry. The models developed have been invaluable for identifying common patterns within a set of structurally diverse molecules with a common mode of action, and have perhaps been even more useful in a practical sense in guiding chemical synthesis of analogs. Although these methods give insight into how well molecules might resemble each other or a composite pharmacophore, the comparisons are largely qualitative, highlighting, for example, where volume is required or excessive in some region. There are no inherent requirements that the molecules be from homologous series, as long as the pharmacophoric elements can be identified in each molecule under consideration. On the contrary, QSAR for the most part is limited to homologous series, and this is a severe limitation when divergent structures form the data set. Since the promise of CoMFA is to advance QSAR beyond this restriction, it is quite natural that these pharmacophore models are typically the starting point for postulating the alignment rule that is so critical to CoMFA. This has been successful in many cases, but it is common in most CoMFA analyses that there are ambiguities in choosing or indeed of finding all of the possibilities for molecular alignment in a given set of molecules. This task is being helped by a number of recently developed automated conformation searching and matching programs. DISCO, a new method for automated pharmacophore generation,[80] is now provided in the SYBYL suite of programs, as is RECEPTOR, a rapid and efficient systematic conformational searching program.[81] Other alignment algorithms which have been used are SEAL[82-87] and SEA4 (QCPE 567).[88] The rapid and automated generation of pharmacophores from a set of structures is an ongoing area of intensive research, and other packages and approaches incorporate a pharmacophore identification step as an integral part of their 3D-QSAR approach (see below). Important studies of alignment questions have been performed on data sets where experimental crystal structure information is available for comparison. These are discussed in detail below.

Other Critical Variables

All of the careful work on CoMFA methodology has pointed out the critical nature of a number of program options to a successful result,[89] and several studies have reported systematic variations of some of these. Important variables that can influence a CoMFA result are grid spacing, orientation of the molecules in the lattice, treatment of field values at boundaries and close to molecules, and statistical treatment of the data. Lattice spacing is typically taken as 2Å, largely for computational efficiency. Many studies have reported that closer spacing does not appear to markedly affect the results. Others have found, however, that simply displacing the lattice by a small amount can markedly affect the results. This observation seems not surprising given the highly nonlinear nature of field isocontours, but is not consistent with the use of a large grid spacing. Folkers et al give a good illustration and discussion of these effects.[89] The bounding region for the analysis is taken as 4Å beyond the union volume of the analysands in all directions. Steric interaction energies become very large close to the van der Waals surface of the molecules, and a constant high value is assigned as a cut-off when this is exceeded. Different cut-off values have been adopted and justified, some preferring the SYBYL default of 30 kcal/mol, but others arguing for a lower value, e.g., 5 kcal/mol. Electrostatic field values between the union volume of all molecules and the van der Waals surface of a particular molecule, i.e., points where the steric energies are assigned the cut-off value, are either set to the average electrostatic value or zero. Scaling of field variables relative to each other and to additional scalar parameters added to the model, e.g., log P, can be critical, especially if variables other than CoMFA fields are included in the model. It is not possible to discuss all of these variations here. Table 5.1 lists some of these issues and selected papers which have studied their variation.

PLS Analysis and Statistical Matters

The statistical technique that makes possible the derivation of a model from so many variables is the partial least squares (PLS) methodology introduced to QSAR by Wold. Descriptions of this procedure are available.[56,135] PLS improves on simple principal components extraction by requiring that the latent variables be constrained to maximally optimize the correlation with the dependent variable as well as be orthogonal to each other. This method uses cross-validation to derive a robust predictive model while also reducing the concern for chance correlations. A study which revisits the approach of Topliss and Edwards to estimating this probability for standard MLR analyses[29] was reported by Cramer for CoMFA-like simulations.[99] It was found that rather low Q^2 values were acceptable for CoMFA analyses without undue concern for chance correlations. The Abbott group makes it a routine practice

Table 5.1. Selected references with informative explorations of CoMFA issues

Issue	References
Options	
grid spacing	86, 89, 90
cutoffs	89, 91, 92
electrostatics treatment	89, 92
lattice displacement	86, 89, 92
scaling	64, 65, 93
Fields	
GRID fields	64, 65, 70, 89, 94
HINT fields	69, 95-97
other fields	
HOMO	78
LUMO	79
MLP	76
scalar variables included	86, 98, 99
indicator variables	98, 100, 101
charge source varied	86, 89
non-standard probes	
(charge = -1)	96, 102, 103
Statistics	
PLS critique	104, 105
GOLPE	70, 106-108
other expimental design	99, 109-112
SAMPLS	83, 113, 114
ACC transforms	90, 115, 116
scrambled data effect	88, 92, 117
Alignment comparison/strategy	78, 90, 91, 98, 102, 103, 118, 119
Interpretation of fields	20, 64, 65, 96, 120
General CoMFA critique	89, 121

Special applications/comparisons

comparison with classical Hansch	94, 99, 120, 122-124
principal properties generation	63, 72, 90, 118, 125-127
steroid binding dataset/	
comparative analyses	18, 32, 66, 69, 83, 109, 128-134

to extract no more than 10 latent variables or 3 less than the number of observations, whichever is less. The choice of the number of latent variables to include is usually based either on the maximum Q^2 or minimum s_{cv}, although other statistics have been championed. For example, Baroni et al propose[107] that SDEP (= PRESS-N) is more suitable as a diagnostic measure of prediction error than SDEC (= s_{cv}). The former statistic is sensitive to the number of cross-validation groups used, increasing as this number decreases.

The PLS analysis is the computationally intensive step of a CoMFA, due both to the large number of variables being processed and the cross-validation procedure which requires the analysis to be repeated. The speed can be improved by prior data reduction using the "minimum sigma" criterion for inclusion of individual grid positions wherein all columns with a standard deviation less than a chosen value are discarded for the cross-validation step. Such points have low variance and only contribute noise to the analysis. In most reported studies, this option causes a substantial reduction in the number of columns to be processed. Another time-saving device is to use a smaller number of cross-validation runs by leaving out more than one compound at a time. Both these devices are applied only at the cross-validation stage, and the final model is run with all columns active. Recent discussions on the effect of noise variables on the ability to uncover significant correlations are focusing more attention on this issue, and some of the statistical design proposals offer alternative possibilities.

Besides these, recent alternatives and improvements to the PLS algorithm itself promise much speedier analyses. The SAMPLS modification[113] recomputes a pairwise covariance matrix between samples (property vectors) and uses this to perform the cross-validation and prediction phases of PLS. This is markedly more efficient computationally while still producing results fully equivalent to standard PLS. Additional benefits in interpretation are outlined by the authors. This program is publicly available (QCPE 650) This method has been proposed recently to be able to take non-linear behavior into account.[114]

There have also been some recent discussions that critically examine just what CoMFA does and does not do.[105] It is frequently claimed that a statistically significant CoMFA provides a relation with "good predictive capability" because of the use of cross-validation. The meaning of this must be carefully understood, however. In fact, this predictability refers to the fact that the derived model is internally consistent, or robust in the statistical sense, and that there are no influential outliers. Where it has been examined, however, the ability of carefully derived CoMFAs to predict beyond the training data set has sometimes been disappointing. One of the main hindrances to understanding the source of this problem is the difficulty of examining the starting parameters for such attributes as range and distribution and frequency of representation in the data set. Issues such as the effect of a large number of "noise" variables have been studied,[104] and the conclusion is that reducing these can lead to better correlations. The CoMFA program as supplied allows data reduction by discarding lattice points with standard deviations less that a specified amount, the minimum sigma option, but the examination of column distributions is not normally possible, and thus one is operating blindly when discarding data points. Data points in a field are not independent and are related in a necessary, continuous manner to adjacent lattice points. This relationship between points will be dependent on the orientation of the molecular set within the grid. Investigations of this continuity question have been reported[115] and a possible solution has been proposed using ACC (auto- and cross-correlation and covariance) transforms. Although these are not firmly established, and are certainly not incorporated into most published CoMFA studies, they offer a promising approach to removing the orientation dependence of results.

A recent paper proposes another method to stabilize CoMFA results to variations in placement within the defined lattice, as well as reducing noise variables.[110] This technique divides the total defined region into 125 subregions and performs 125 analyses, one for each region. Regions which give a Q^2 greater than a predefined amount (the authors used a generous cutoff of 0.0) were retained and combined to form a reduced operational region to be used in the actual analysis. This had the effect of reducing the dimensionality and "noise" variables as well as largely eliminating the sensitivity of Q^2 to orientation within the region. Consistently better models were obtained for previously published analyses.

The question of experimental design for CoMFA studies has been investigated. Unfortunately, the usual method of finding a sparse set of well distributed parameters and observations with which to derive a model is not consistent with the cross-validation approach of the PLS methodology, and, given the highly nonlinear nature of fields, perhaps not even suitable. The GOLPE method has been examined as a way of deriving the most robust model from the available data by introducing a D-optimal design step at the latent factor extraction stage with the intent of amplifying the signal-to-noise ratio.[70,106-108,136] Improvement in the models examined was observed. True experimental design would require the ability to examine the distribution and intercorrelation of the independents and then add or select additional examples to optimize the former and minimize the latter. This is virtually impossible for the raw variables in CoMFA (and probably not even desirable), but design in the latent variables as is done in GOLPE is the reasonable alternative. Although the latent variables may be examined for distributional characteristics, it is not at all evident how to devise a compound or compounds that rectify imbalances. This difficulty is exacerbated by the variable practices of handling steric cutoffs and electrostatics between the union volume of the set and the van der Waals volume of a given molecule. Additionally, there would be a need to chose analogs that would maintain sufficient variability to prevent points from being excluded by the minimum sigma criterion. The commercial version of COMFA does not allow the easy examination of the composition of extracted latent variables; other implementations generally do. Factorial design has been examined in a study of α-chymotrypsin inhibitors.[111] Another approach from the same group[112] used cluster analysis of principal components derived from CoMFA energy descriptors to select a training set from a large collection of analogs.

The true test of any QSAR model, 2D or 3D, is whether it can predict the activity of compounds not used to derive the model. This has always been the weak link in reported retrospective QSAR studies. Will the model predict the activity of compounds it should predict, i.e., those within the parameter space of the training set, and how far beyond those boundaries is it useful? In CoMFA, unlike QSAR, the parameter space is not easily available for inspection. The commercial program provides a warning when pre-diction compounds have unique features not found in the training set, but it takes a painstaking analysis to understand where these points are. If one takes statistical strictures at face value, the promise of CoMFA to deal effectively with non-homologous sets of mole-cules is thus vitiated. Features that may markedly enhance or di-minish activity may be just those regions in pharmacophore mod-els which extend differentially beyond the union volume. One has only to look at the rationalizations of inactivity advanced from active-analog-derived pharmacophore models to appreciate that "re-ceptor required volume" appears at diverse points around a union volume, and that each inactive analog often seems to protrude into its own unique space.

There are several aspects of validation that can be identified for CoMFA models. The first hurdle, of course, is to obtain a significant model. If this can be accomplished, the question then arises whether this is the best possible model. Work reported with GOLPE and the recent report on reduced region identification[110] has pointed the direction to obtaining consistent and stable CoMFA models, but has also shown that the standard implementation may miss significant models or produce sub-optimal models if care is not taken to investigate different option settings. This particularly illustrates the danger of relying on the results obtained using only the default settings provided in the commercial program. Beyond obtaining a robust model, however, is the ability of the model to predict compounds not used in its derivation. For example, a CoMFA analysis might be expected to be able to validate at least the main features of an existing pharmacophore model. The se-quence of papers on angiotensin converting enzyme (ACE) inhibi-tors reported from the Washington University group[78,98,137,138] are particularly valuable in understanding the strengths and limitations of CoMFA models in a situation where no receptor structure is available. A comprehensive pharmacophore model covering several classes of ACE inhibitor and according well with the extensive body of medicinal and biochemical knowledge had been derived. Ini-tially "acceptable" CoMFA models performed much more poorly than expected on predicting new compounds, especially for cer-tain subsets. A number of attempts to improve or rectify the situation were examined, including varying program options, investigating more rigorously determined charge sets, and adding additional variables for flexibility and other effects. The final conclusion was that all of the subtypes of inhibitor could not be included in the same model, the sulfhydryl subset being the worst behaved. Separate models for individual classes, however, performed in a much more consistent manner.

Another set of papers which are instructive in this regard are the studies performed on ligands for the benzodiazepine receptors. Several successful CoMFA studies have now been reported for ligands of this receptor and there begins to be the opportunity for the "lateral validation" of QSARs as advocated by Hansch.[139] Unlike the ACE work, these studies have come from different laboratories.[73,136,140-142] Here, not only are at least five CoMFA studies available, but there have been several pharmacophore models proposed and extensive classical QSAR work on various subseries. In addition, a distance geometry study[143] and a MSA study[35] are available. Hansch has included discussion of some of this work in his extensive review of benzodiazepine QSAR[144] and Zhang et al[145] include this in their review of pharmacophore modeling. Both discussions show how CoMFA results can be used to support an existing body of work.

It has been stressed that a CoMFA model, in the absence of a receptor structure, should not be taken to be a receptor map,[89] any more so than is a pharmacophore model. CoMFA nonetheless has a unique opportunity to be tested for the adequacy of its assumptions when experimental structural information is available. Increasingly the crystal structures of series of compounds bound to the same macromolecule are becoming available. To the degree that these can be accepted as bona fide bound conformations, an experimentally verified alignment is thereby obtained, and the contribution of this difficult matter to the success of the analysis can be fixed. Several detailed studies have appeared on such data sets, and the results are illuminating and sobering. A set of anti-rhinoviral oxazolines is notorious for illustrating the danger of assuming a common binding mode for apparently similar congeners.[146] Rossmann et al demonstrated by crystallographic studies that these molecules can adopt two distinct active site binding

modes which are inversely related to each other.[147] An initial
CoMFA was reported on this data set by Diana et al[148-150] which,
however, did not address this key feature in any depth. Analysis
of this same set as part of a critical evaluation of CoMFA assumptions by Klebe et al[91] came to the disturbing conclusion that a
deliberately incorrect, but intuitive, alignment of the molecules,
gave a CoMFA result statistically equivalent to that obtained with
the experimentally found alignment. Evidently, standard CoMFA
fields are unable to distinguish subtle, though clearly critical, variations in molecular properties determining binding. In a second
study on thermolysin inhibitors, it was found that alignments based
on reasonable superposition rules and energy minimization and/or
field fitting, gave higher Q^2 than those derived directly from the
crystal structures. The Washington University group did additional
work on the thermolysin set, trying additional indicator parameters for Zn ligand type to improve the fit as was tried in the
ACE study.[78] In this case no benefit was observed. In both
thermolysin studies, the data set is a mixture of actual crystal structures and analogs of related compounds modeled on the closest
available experimental structure, so the data is a mixture of actual
and modeled structures. A further study of this data set using a
new variant of the CoMFA method, comparative molecular similarity analysis (CoMSIA),[83] (see below), has also obtained similar
results using an alternate alignment method and field description.

In a series of papers from the Washington University group,
inhibitors of HIV protease have been analyzed. These are highly
flexible peptide-like molecules similar in kind to the thermolysin
inhibitors. Crystal structures of prototype compounds for five different bioisostere series were used to model additional analogs in
each series. Five different alignment rules were examined in the
first paper,[102] the best being based on field-fitting each modeled
compound onto the crystal conformation of its prototype. Additionally, an alignment based on minimization of each ligand in
the enzyme active site was examined, as well as variants of these
which included charged and ionized side chains. The first alignment gave the best results, both for model Q^2 and predictive ability outside the training set on molecules from yet another
bioisostere series. A second paper[103] proposed a method, NewPred,

to examine more than one possible alignment for prediction set molecules in order to consider alternative binding modes. The third paper examined in more detail the CoMFA fields from predictive models with respect to the ligand binding site of the enzyme to determine the degree to which CoMFA contours can be matched with receptor features.[96] The latter paper tried adding HINT fields, but did not find them to be helpful for this series of compounds. The CoMSIA study of this data set claimed improved interpretability and correspondence with enzyme features.[83]

Carrieri et al[122] used CoMFA to support results of a classical QSAR study on papain substrates. A conclusion from classical QSAR that meta substituents should be oriented differently, depending on their hydrophobic character, was confirmed. In this case, since no hydrophobic fields were used, the combination of favorable and unfavorable steric and electrostatic CoMFA regions were equated with the hydrophobic effects found in the classical QSAR. Greco et al in their study of a variable selection procedure[99] made reference to the enzyme cavity to assess the validity of their CoMFA model. Here also a classical QSAR provided the background for the study. A study using GRID fields in an evaluation of the GOLPE method also used crystal data for the glycogen phosphorylase *b* active site to evaluate the results of various CoMFA runs.[70]

CoMFA Application Survey

Publications on CoMFA continue to appear at an increasing rate. Many of these, unfortunately, simply use the default settings and recommendations given in the SYBYL documentation, and many of the same questions and problems cling to these studies that are characteristic of "turn the crank" QSAR analyses in general. Especially in assessing applications for whether the CoMFA method makes sense in the terms that it is formulated, there is frequently uncritical acceptance. As will be seen below, the reporting of conditions of the analysis is very uneven, and frequently, insufficient detail about how the analysis was run is provided for proper evaluation. Recommendations for reporting CoMFA results have been published in at least two places,[151,152] and it is strongly urged that the information suggested to be included in these guidelines be provided by authors and insisted upon by editors and reviewers of CoMFA contributions. This being noted, many "successful" CoMFA analyses have been reported in a wide variety of situations. These are collected below in several categories.

Physical Property Estimation

CoMFA has been examined for its ability to provide an alternate method for calculating various physical properties. This would be of utility where estimates are needed of difficult to obtain or measure compounds. Waller[97] reported that CoMFA may be used to estimate log Ps for a congeneric series of halogenated aromatic hydrocarbons. The method was able to improve on the calculation by the CLOGP program[153] by taking account of positional effects. A combination of CoMFA and HINT fields was found to be best in correlating two sets of data, HPLC retention time and measured log P. Norinder has reported the use of steric and electrostatic fields to generate principal properties to serve as theoretical descriptors of nucleic acid bases for QSAM (quantitative sequence activity models).[126] A similar application of this approach had been reported earlier to generate principal properties for amino acid side chains using fields for steric, electrostatic and lipophilic character.[63] A different set of principal properties for amino acid side chains were derived using six GRID fields by Cocchi and Johansson.[72] Kim and Martin[62,114] evaluated CoMFA for estimating Hammett substituent constants, and Norinder has used his modification of CoMFA to generate a set of principal properties for aromatic substituents.[125] van de Waterbeemd has also investigated the use of CoMFA for this purpose.[90,118] In the latter case, the hope was that this would be a convenient source of parameters for unusual substituents. This author discusses several operational problems with this superficially attractive idea and concludes, with Norinder above, that this has no advantage over direct CoMFA analysis on a given problem.

Related to these studies aimed at using CoMFA or field-based models to generate or estimate physical or reactivity properties are the studies which apply CoMFA to previously existing Hansch correlations. A summary of CoMFA correlations with all of the standard Hansch, Hammett and Taft parameters has been given by Kim.[123] Kim has also published a series of studies using his GRID/CoMFA method to systematically compare the ability of various GRID fields to reproduce biological Hansch QSARs which were based on single properties, specifically, lipophilicity (log P or π, both linear and parabolic), electronic (σ) and steric (E_s) parameters. In all cases correlations as good as the original based on substituent effect parameters were obtained. The data sets were carefully chosen so that only single properties were the determinant of activity. Hydrophobic effects within series were well represented by GRID fields using a water probe[154] Another recent application reports the correlation of reversed phase HPLC capacity factors for sets of simply substituted pyrazines and pyridines using only a water probe.[155] Fields generated with the H^+ probe were found to reproduce correlations with the Hammett σ parameters and related variants.[156,157] It is interesting that, while the standard σ and the inductive component of this, $\mathfrak{I}$ or σ_I, were well correlated by CoMFA using a proton probe, the resonance component, $\mathfrak{R}$, did not fare as well. Evidently, the pi polarization implicit in $\mathfrak{R}$ is not well reflected in the projected fields probed by a proton probe. Correlations with parameters σ^+ or σ^- where this effect is maximized were not reported, although QSARs containing these terms were reproduced by GRID/CoMFA models. For steric parameters, good representations of surface area and volume were possible with the steric probe.[157,158] MR, MW and υ, Charton's steric parameter, all appear to contain additional information not captured by this probe. For E_s the combination of a steric and electrostatic field seemed to give the best result, though no discussion was offered of the extent to which the model might be fitting experimental error, in spite of the supporting statistics.

These studies are very useful in illustrating (a) the extent to which CoMFA derived latent variables mimic well understood physical chemical substituent effects and (b) where they may diverge and offer different information. These findings raise an interesting question of interpretation. Does the regionalization of property variation imposed by the CoMFA methodology have independent validity; and give additional insight into the actual interactions involved or is this equivalence a statistical artifact giving spurious implications of local effects? Conversely, the Hansch parameters could be serving as surrogates for local interactions if the CoMFA view is taken to be true. Charton has frequently argued that interpretation is most informative when "pure effect" parameters are used and more problematical when "mixed effect" parameters, log P for example, are used,[159] especially if intermolecular interactions are being studied. At present it does not seem possible to tell when CoMFA is modeling a regional effect and when it is partitioning a global one. Other comparison studies between Hansch and CoMFA on the same data sets are discussed below, some of which give a little more insight on this issue.

A recent CoMFA study was able to correlate both log D and solubilities of amino acids.[160] Again, GRID fields from a water probe were sufficient to correlate log D with three components for a mixture of 38 free and N-acetyl-aminoacid amides. For solubility, a two component model using both a water and the CoMFA electrostatic probe gave the best result. CoMFA-derived principal properties of heterocycles have been applied by Langer.[127]

All of the above suggests that CoMFA might be used to generate "missing" parameters for standard MLR or in cases where ambiguity complicates assignment of these, as for example in using heterocycles in a set of substituted benzene analogs. van de Waterbeemd[90] concluded that, at least for complex groups, conformational multiplicity limited the usefulness of such methods. A similar concern was observed in the generation of amino acid side chain parameters. The CoMFA latent variables contain much of the same information present in other parameters but in different combinations. The degree to which minor components reflect specific adjustments for particular functional groups does not seem to have been reported. The other difficulty with this approach is that new parameters require local generation of the CoMFA model and thus use of data reported in the literature cannot be easily extended to new groups which may be of interest.

Additional studies using CoMFA to correlate physical properties are instructive. Kim and Martin extended their work on correlating benzoic acid acidity (and consequently Hammett σ values)[62] to the estimation of the pK_a of clonidine derivatives.[161] The success of this is promising, since ortho substituents are prominent in this data set, a group that is not well handled by simple parameterization. A CoMFA study was used to develop a predictive model for the transport of a diverse set of aromatic molecules through polydimethylsiloxane membranes.[162] Best results required the addition of scalar terms for hydrophobicity (f_{chex}), solubility and indicators for ring systems and intramolecular H-bonding. Apparently the steric and electrostatic fields of CoMFA alone are not able to adequately account for these effects. A CoMFA/HINT study of host/guest complexes of a series of barbiturates with α- and β-cyclodextrins[95] reported that CoMFA gave adequate correlations for both sets and HINT added little. Given the nature of the substructures involved, this is not surprising since they are all contain alkyl groups in the variable portion and the steric and hydrophobic fields contain much of the same information.

BIOLOGICAL DATA SETS

The number of reported CoMFA studies is increasing rapidly. In some biological systems it is possible to examine the reported CoMFA studies in the spirit of the comparative QSAR approach of Hansch[130] with the expectation that relationships in similar systems might share similar features. Selected reported studies have been grouped below for comment by type of biological target.

GPCR Ligands

Quite a few studies have been reported on ligands for the G-protein coupled receptor (GPCR) family of transmembrane receptors. Ligands for these receptors are important drugs and the receptors of the family are important targets for many current therapeutic strategies. Since the biological data for such studies are primarily from receptor binding assays, it should be of the precision needed to give good correlations. These cannot all be discussed here, but a summary of CoMFA results on these and closely related ligands is given in Table 5.2 to facilitate comparison.

Generalizations are difficult due to the wide variation in reporting of details of the analyses, but one common theme is the great predominance of the steric field as the primary determinant of activity. The level of precision achieved by these correlations tends to be only modest, but in several cases, examples have been given of the heuristic value of the derived models either in predicting analogs outside the training set or in "prescreening" synthesis proposals. Most of the reported analyses use only the standard CoMFA fields. A description by Martin[163] of the evolution of a CoMFA model over time for dopamine D1 receptors is especially instructive in showing what may be expected from this approach, and its use for analyzing such important questions as specificity is illustrated. Another study of note in this table is that of Agarwal and Taylor.[170] Here CoMFA was used to correlate intrinsic activity, as opposed to affinity. A pharmacophore model including both agonists and antagonists was successfully constructed. Whether 3D-QSAR methods will be up to the challenge of providing convincing alignment rules for the diverse structures that bind well to this family of important receptors remains to be determined.

Ion Channel Modulators

Compounds interacting with ion-channels of various types have been studied with CoMFA. The benzodiazepine receptor was one of the first to be successfully subjected to CoMFA.[136,181] Another analysis on a different set of compounds has also been reported with similar good results.[141] Kim et al have compared the GRID/CoMFA approach to the standard SYBYL/CoMFA approach for a large set of benzodiazepines from an earlier combined QSAR/CoMFA study.[73] This study is one of the first to directly compare these variants. Although results of similar quality and predictive capability were obtained for both the SYBYL/CoMFA and the GRID/CoMFA, problems reconciling the interpretation of the derived models were noted.

A brief report of an application to potassium channel openers compares CoMFA with a traditional QSAR at a single position.[182] The CoMFA replicates the accompanying Hansch analysis, although both seem to be statistically over-determined.

A study of the binding of the natural product ryanodine and analogs to the vertebrate skeletal muscle ryanodine receptor used CoMFA to derive details of the binding interaction.[183] Unfortunately, no details of the analysis are included for proper evaluation.

Inhibitors of the astrocytic chloride channel were studied by both conventional QSAR and CoMFA with similar good models

Table 5.2. CoMFA studies of GPCR and related ligands

Ref.	Activity/Compound class	Align	Charges†	N	Q^2 (comp)	S_{cv}	R^2	Steric/Elec‡	Other†	Comparison	Comment
163	D1 ligands, agonist, antagonists, binding, function mixed types	DISCO	nr					only steric	GRID/CoMFA	CoMFA adjunct to pharmaco-phore model	sequential development over time of models; only steric fields important
164	D1 antagonists, binding pKi, SCH23390 analogs	field	DelRe	12 11	0.46(4) 0.58(2)	1.09 0.72	0.99 0.99	nr	+ torsion angle term	conventional QSAR with dipole vector and torsion angle, $R^2 = 0.92$; see also ref 165	field fit much better than rms on pharmacophore; CoMFA details sparse
125	D2 antagonists, binding pIC50, benzamides	rms	nr	70	0.72(4)		0.85	nr	not SYBYL CoMFA fields	comparison to standard QSAR ref 166	evaluation of 3D-PP descriptors for substituents vs standard Hansch parameters
167	D2 antagonists, binding log(IC50), clozapine analogs	rms	nr	38	0.31(6)	0.86	0.96	0.56/0.44			CoMFA details sparse

168	5HT1a, binding pKi, arylpiperazines	rms	gast/huck	50	0.68(3)	0.89	0.47/0.53		20 additional analogs predicted with reasonable accuracy
93	5HT1a, binding pKi, arylpiperazines	rms	AM1?	43	0.78(3)	0.92	0.53/0.47 (CoMFA std scaling); 0.98/0.02 (no scaling)	3 alignment variations examined	randomizing method used to check chance correlation; steric field only gives $Q^2 = 0.86(3)$
169	5HT1a, 5HT1b antagonists, binding, phenoxypropanol amines	multifit + field	nr	17	?(5) (both subtypes)	0.99 (both subtypes)	0.92/0.08 (both subtypes)	CoMFA adjunct to pharmacophore model	CoMFA details very sparse
170	5HT1a, intrinsic activity, mixed types	rms	MNDO	20	0.48(5)	0.94	0.94/0.06	CoMFA adjunct to pharmacophore model	intrinsic activity of mixed type with common alignment of agonists and antagonists, CoMFA details sparse
171	5HT1a, 5HT2, binding pKi, tetrahydropyridinyl-indoles	rms	MNDO	45	0.45(4) (5HT1a) 0.41(5) (5HT2)	0.85 (1a) 0.84 (2)	0.87/0.13 (1a) 0.76/0.24 (2)	conventional QSAR on subset; ref 172	6 additional analogs well predicted, CoMFA details sparse Compass analysis on 5HT1a affinity, ref 226

Table 5.2. CoMFA studies of GPCR and related ligands (continued)

Ref.	Activity/ Compound class	Align	Charges†	N	Q^2 (comp)	S_{cv}	R^2	Steric/ Elec‡	Other†	Comparison	Comment
173	muscarinic agonists, pD2, rat jejunum, mixed types	rms	gast	39	0.71(4)	0.42	0.90	nr	AM1 charge set also examined	CoMFA adjunct to pharmacophore model	5 models examined with different options
76	alpha1, binding pKi, pyrazolopyridines;	1) atom rms	gast	38	0.76(5)		0.92 with	steric only	MLP field examined studied standard		utility of MLP field
	alpha1, binding pIC50, mixed types	2) atom rms		33	0.58(7)		0.84 only	MLP	CoMFA		
71	alpha1 antagonists, binding, prazosin analogs			14	0.73 (2)	0.11 (SDEC) 0.32 (SDEP)	0.96	nr	GRID/ GOLPE		CoMFA details very sparse, H_2O and aromatic CH GRID probes gave similar contours
174	histamine H1 antagonists, pA2, thiazolidin-4-ones	rms	MNDO	15	0.55(3)	0.82	0.91	nr		conventional QSAR with 3 Hansch parmeters	Hansch analysis on same set gave $R^2 = 0.80$, s = 0.54, CoMFA details sparse

				n					CoMFA role	Comments
35	CCK-A antagonists, binding log(IC50) benzodiazepines	field	gast	18	0.45(5) (9cv groups)		0.99	nr	CoMFA adjunct to pharmacophore model	CoMFA details very sparse F_{cv} doesn't reach significance (p = 0.16), MSA analysis on similar set ref 175
176	CCK-B antagonists, binding pIC50, benzodiazepines	atom rms	gast/ huck	20 (19)	0.57(5) (0.87(5))	0.92 (0.51)	0.99	nr	CoMFA adjunct to pharmacophore model	12 additional compounds predicted with mixed success
82	AT1 antagonists, binding p(IC50), biphenyls (mixed acid isosteres)	SEAL	MNDO	50	0.64(2)	0.66	0.75	nr	CoMFA adjunct to pharmacophore model	39 additional compounds predicted with overall good success
117	ETa inhibitors, pIC50 for binding, isoxazole sulfonamides	rms	PM3	32	0.58(5)	0.80	0.94 0.70/	ca "simple" charge set adjunct to 0.30 examined, several alignments tried	CoMFA activities used pharmacophore model	scrambled as check for chance correlation, CoMFA used to choose best alignment

Table 5.2. CoMFA studies of GPCR and related ligands (continued)

Ref.	Activity/ Compound class	Align	Charges†	N	Q² (comp)	S_{cv}	R²	Steric/ Elec‡	Other†	Comparison	Comment
119	GH releasing activity, -log (rel pot), somat-ostatin analogs	1) rms	Pullman	64	0.51(5)	0.54 (1.02 SDEP)	0.86	0.61/ 0.39	several alignments tried		comparison of different models for true pre-dictive capability
		2) field			0.57(5)	0.40 (0.95 SDEP)	0.92	0.62/0.38			
		3) pharma-ophore			0.55(5)	0.50 (0.98 SDEP)	0.98	0.61/0.39			
177	cannabinoid, pIC50 for binding, ED50s in 4 functional assays, THC analogs	rms	nr	33	0.31(4) (binding) 0.50-0.65(5) (function)		0.96 (binding) 0.88-0.91 (function)	ca. 0.40/0.60			CoMFA details very sparse, results for behavioral tests better than for binding data
178	sigma, binding pKi, mixed types	rms	gast	31	0.84(4)	0.52	0.98	0.93/0.07		CoMFA adjunct to pharmacophore model	predictions outside training set from literature sources, 36 additional analogs with good overall predictability

179	sigma3 agonists, binding pIC50, mixed types	DISCO + field	gast	34	0.61(5)	0.73	0.94	0.70/ 0.30	CoMFA adjunct to pharmacophore model	some compounds excluded for poor fit, molecules protonated
180	sigma1, binding pKi, normetazocine analogs	nr	nr	19	0.39			nr	HINT	standard QSAR gave better result $R^2 = 0.90$	CoMFA details very sparse, HINT offered no improvement

† abbreviations: nr = not reported; rms = root mean square fit on selected atoms or pharmacophore elements; field = field fit; gast (/huck) = Gasteiger/ (Hückel); Q^2 = cross-validated R^2; s_{cv} = cross validation standard error of estimate (= SDEC); SDEP = standard error of prediction; comp = number of latent variables.

‡ relative contribution of steric and electrostatic fields to CoMFA model.

arising.[184] The conventional QSAR included dipole moment and CLOGP as parameters. CoMFA for four alignments gave similar results with two to three components. The composition of the CoMFA terms was not reported.

The combination of six structural classes of compounds which block the GABA receptor at the picrotoxin site were studied.[88] In spite of the fact that all are noncompetitive inhibitors, it was possible to combine them into a single analysis with a Q^2 of 0.45. Randomization of the dependent variable was used as a check against chance correlation. SEA4 was used to align the rather diverse structures and Gasteiger charges were employed.

Calcium channel agonists were studied by Davis et al[64,65,185] using GRID fields processed by the PLS routine in SIMCA 4.4.[186] This study is of note because the authors graphically examined the contributions of the individual latent variables to determine both the regions represented by each component and the steric and electronic field points giving similar information. This looks to be a very useful way to get at least a peek into the "black box" of the standard composite CoMFA fields. A CoMFA analysis of 5HT3 arylpiperazines has been reported.[187]

Enzymes

Folkers et al have stated[89] that enzyme/substrate interactions should provide the best data for CoMFA, or indeed any QSAR, analyses. Some of the most careful and comprehensive studies of the CoMFA methodology have utilized enzyme inhibition data, both without (ACE inhibitors) and with (thermolysin inhibitors, HIV protease inhibitors) ancillary crystal structure information (see above). These studies especially illustrate the care and effort that is needed to obtain consistent and sensible CoMFA models, and suggest that many of the simplifying assumptions of the COMFA technique are inadequate. The results tend to give only modest "goodness of fit" statistics (Q^2 = 0.4-0.7 and R^2 = 0.7-0.9) in the best cases. There seem to be no general procedures that can be relied upon to extract the "best model" and sensitivity to method options varies greatly from one analysis to another. For this reason, reported analyses which do not give evidence of having explored these variations must remain suspect in spite of being formally acceptable by the PLS cross-validation criterion. Certainly interpretations based on such models are likely to be without merit. Other enzyme applications besides those already discussed above under validation issues include DHFR inhibitors,[99,101] α-chymotrypsin,[111,112] prolyl endopeptidase inhibitors,[188] ACAT inhibitors,[189] HMG CoA reductase inhibitors,[190] thermitase,[191] MAO inhibitors[192] and HIV integrase inhibitors.[92] The latter study examined the variation of several CoMFA options including lattice placement and electrostatics treatment.

Other Binding Data

Cocaine analogs inhibiting the dopamine transporter have been the most studied of this group.[49,124,193] These studies report parallel classical Hansch analyses. The initial study found CoMFA to provide a model where standard Hansch analysis failed. Follow-up work was reported in the latter study which casts some question on the predictive utility of the original model. This data set was also subjected to analysis by the Voronoi binding site method.[46] Comparison of conclusions between the two methods is not straightforward. Good et al also examined this data set as part of their evaluation of a similarity-based alternative to CoMFA (see below).[132]

The original CoMFA correlated the binding of steroids to steroid binding globulin.[18] This data set has become a benchmark for newly proposed 3D-QSAR techniques and it has been reanalyzed now by quite a number of methods. These are collected in Table 5.1. A similar set of molecules binding to androgen or progestin receptors was reported.[194] For progestins, steric fields were superior to combined or standard QSAR parameters. For androgens, methodological difficulties prevented the proper assessment of an apparent electrostatic contribution. CoMFA was also used to correlate receptor binding activities of chlorinated estradiol derivatives to the estrogen receptor.[195]

A study of the binding of taxol derivatives to microtubules gave equivalent models with either steric, electrostatic or both fields.[196] The model was applied to an extensive prediction set. Several low actives were not well predicted. Some of these would appear to extend beyond the region sampled by the training set.

Interaction of anti-HIV porphorins with gp120 envelope glycoprotein were studied with CoMFA.[197]

Cellular and In Vivo Activity

Two papers were published by Horwitz et al reporting successful CoMFA analyses of the growth inhibition activity of pyrazolo [3,4,5-kl]acridine intercalators against two tumor cell lines in vitro.[85] CoMFA models, though "successful" were unable to rationalize the selectivity of compounds toward L1210 and HCT-8 cells. A second study of 9H-thioxanthen-9-ones against pancreatic ductal adenocarcinoma, a solid tumor, in vivo[86] examined variations in charge calculation method, lattice spacing and offset and charge state of the molecules, as well as additional scalar parameters to arrive at a final CoMFA model. SEAL was used for alignment.

A successful CoMFA model of the relative antimalarial activity of artemisinin analogs was obtained.[198] The relative steric/electronic contributions were 0.66/0.34 in the final model. This model was able to successfully predict the activity of 14 additional compounds of varied structure and a broad range of activity.

Induction of human leukemia cell differentiation by alkyl amides was examined by CoMFA.[199] The predictive capability of this model was only moderate for new analogs.

Agricultural Chemistry

New applications to compounds of agricultural interest have been reported. Both the study on knockdown activity of pyrethroids[200] and that on anilide inhibitors of the Hill reaction[201] sought to use CoMFA to replace steric terms in a traditional Hansch equation with CoMFA field terms. Both found CoMFA to be successful in this regard.

Toxicological Applications

Mutagenicity of chlorinated hydroxyfuranones, previously correlated with E_{lumo} was re-examined in CoMFA and an attempt was made to utilize the LUMO orbital.[79] E_{lumo} continued to be the primary determinant of activity with a questionable improvement by the CoMFA steric fields.

A study of the toxicity of chlorophenols to *Photobacterium phosphoreum* gave a result with CoMFA that showed steric fields able to accommodate the reduced toxicity of 2,6-substituted analogs better that a simple log P correlation.[202] The exact nature of the effect as steric or electronic was not unambiguous. Although the steric field gave a higher R^2 than the electrostatic field when taken individually, both were within the limits of the experimental error.

Comparison with Traditional QSAR

Several papers have reported comparisons of Hansch analyses with CoMFA. These give various assessments of the complementarity and mutual interpretability of the results from the two approaches. A study of genotoxic nitrofurans illustrates some difficulties in cross-interpretation between the methods.[120] Similar ambiguities were observed in the study of papain catalyzed hydrolysis of aryl esters cited earlier.[122] Improved correlations using a combined Hansch/CoMFA approach were reported for anilide inhibitors of the Hill reaction.[201] Other examples where the methods have been compared have been discussed above. A selection of these is included in Table 5.1. Many of the 3D-QSAR studies were performed without using hydrophobic fields. Much of the discussion on comparative interpretation of the models centers on the inadequacy of standard CoMFA to reproduce the hydrophobic effect with only steric and electrostatic fields.

SIMILARITY METHODS

A second very active line of research that has provided an alternate to the CoMFA perspective on the problem of 3D-QSAR encompasses the efforts to devise and manipulate measures of molecular similarity.[203-207] These include a number of mathematical and statistical approaches to compare molecules quantitatively for similarity based on topological or field-type information. Several of these similarity methods have been proposed as alternative 3D-QSAR approaches to CoMFA. MSA, discussed above was an early example of this approach in a QSAR setting. Unlike CoMFA which considers every point in a grid sampling of a field as an independent parameter to be evaluated in a linear model, similarity methods make use of a similarity function to derive a pairwise "distance" measure between two compounds. For a set of N compounds, an N x N matrix of pairwise similarities is generated.

Many different functions have been devised for this purpose[128,131,132,208-215] using field, topological, or physicochemical properties as a basis. Their use in QSAR, though growing, is much more limited at this point, and experience is correspondingly less as to their general utility. Some of the more interesting and promising of these are mentioned here.

Good et al reanalyzed the steroid binding data used by Cramer in his original CoMFA paper using neural network pattern recognition on a full similarity matrix based on both shape similarity and electrostatic similarity. A QSAR of comparable quality was obtained and computational efficiency was much higher.[128] A follow-up paper evaluated different similarity functions and utilized the GOLPE method to optimize model derivation. Several additional data sets of different sorts were studied. Results were frequently better than the comparable CoMFA analyses.[132] This method lacks the interpretive aids of CoMFA field contouring, however. Use of a similarity approach to treat chirality was illustrated.[216] Using the shape similarity function employed in the above studies to generate a single variable based on comparisons with two reference molecules gave a QSAR reminiscent of MSA for a set of dihydrofolate reductase (DHFR) inhibitors.[217] Previous analysis of this set by classical QSAR methods yielded a six-parameter equation. Interestingly, three subseries gave different correlation equations. Similarly, five- or six-parameter Hansch equations for the hypotensive activity of 27 clonidine analogs could be replaced with relation using a single similarity index. The resulting equation, though of similar statistical quality to the more complex expression, proved to have improved predictive ability as judged by the cross-validation criterion.

Benigni et al have recently reported a closer analysis of how two frequently used similarity indices, the Carbo and Hodgkin indices, perform in relation to physicochemical parameters for a discriminant analysis of mutation induction by halogenated aliphatic hydrocarbons.[218] It was found that the information content of the similarity matrices was similar to that of the property matrix, but that, even though discriminants of similar quality could be obtained, no improvement was obtained on combining the two types. For this data set, the shape information inherent in the simi-

larity measures did not add to that already in the property parameters, several of which were of a geometric nature.

Very recently, an approach to combining similarity ideas and
methods within the CoMFA framework, Comparative Molecular
Similarity Analysis (CoMSIA), was reported.[83] Field values at the
lattice points are redefined as similarities to a probe with a particular physical property; summed over all atoms in the molecule.
Steric, electrostatic and hydrophobic property fields were generated by interaction with a CoMFA-like probe having radius 1Å,
charge +1 and hydrophobicity +1. Corresponding atomic properties were the third power of the atomic radius, atomic partial
charge, obtained in the usual way, and the atomic hydrophobicity
contributions devised by Viswanadhan et al.[219] The preferred alignment was by obtained using SEAL.[84,87] Analyses of the steroid data
set used by Cramer[18] as a relatively rigid, homologous series, and
the thermolysin inhibitors studied by DePriest[98] as a flexible, diverse
series with crystallographic data, both gave models of comparable
numerical quality to the original CoMFAs. The contour maps.
showed localized maxima much more in character and conjunction
with corresponding enzyme binding functional groups. This was
especially apparent in matching features of the CoMSIA map with
the corresponding regions of the thermolysin crystal structure. This
promising method also purports to resolve some of the mathematical and theoretical issues with the CoMFA field properties.

HASL

Several papers have now appeared on another grid-based approach called HASL (Hypothetical Active Site Lattice).[220-222] This
method, which has some kinship to the MTD approach, uses a
cubic lattice in just the converse sense to CoMFA to provide a
simplified representation of the shape and properties of a molecule, as opposed to the region around it. A lattice representation
is prepared for each molecule in a set and the lattice points are
assigned the properties of the nearest atom. As in CoMFA, different lattice spacing may be examined. The lattice points are then
fit using a simple optimizing function to build up a composite
lattice sequentially, adding one compound at a time. A HASL
model results which best fits the whole data set. This provides a

superposition hypothesis for the set. For QSAR, activity values are partitioned among the lattice points by an interactive process. New compounds are predicted by fitting them to the lattice and adding the activity contributions of the points in common. In spite of the rather simple molecular representation, sensible results and modest predictions have been obtained. Recent improvements have addressed matters of computational efficiency and statistical robustness.[222-224]

OTHER METHODS

A number of other novel approaches to incorporating the third dimension into QSAR have been reported recently. These often combine a pharmacophore identification and activity estimation phase as illustrated by HASL. COMPASS[129,225,226] generates a shape-based molecular description which concentrates on the surface properties of compounds. A set of property vectors extending beyond the van der Waals surface are associated with each conformer of each molecule. A neural network is then trained to simultaneously predict activity as a function of the features and, also, for each molecule, choose the conformation which is the bioactive one. This method gave better performance on the benchmark steroid data set of Cramer than either the original CoMFA or the similarity analyses previously mentioned. Another surface-based approach is the recently reported Receptor Surface Model (RSM).[133,227] A hypothetical receptor surface complementary to the union of a set of active analogs is created and steric and electrostatic properties are deduced and mapped onto this surface. An energy of interaction is calculated for each ligand of interest and this, along with an internal strain energy term are used to seek a correlation with relative affinity. The benchmark steroid data set was also examined by this method. The RSM method makes less of a point about statistical purity and seems to be aimed at being a flexible hypothesis generating tool. A Genetic Function Algorithm[228] is used to find alternative models.

Other groups have reported novel approaches to 3D-QSAR, but discussion of these is beyond the scope of this review. Some of the more interesting are the work of Belvisi et al using a novel chemometric approach to identify bioactive conformers,[229-231] the "heuristic-direct" approach of the de Benedetti group to use calculated binding energies of ligands with receptor models,[232-234] and Mager's processing of molecular Cartesian coordinates by multivariate analysis.[235,236]

For situations where the structures of both ligand and receptor are available, correlation of binding energies calculated from modeled receptor ligand complexes is perhaps the most direct approach to 3D-QSAR. Direct estimation of binding energies with adequate reliability and precision is still very difficult. Some recent reports of success in this approach[237,238] suggest that this goal may be closer than we think.

Finally, there are a number of new methods embodied in commercial software packages which utilize proprietary approaches to 3D-QSAR, usually in the context of a suite of programs designed for drug design. Unfortunately, not all of these are adequately documented in the open literature to date, and it is not possible to properly assess their validity, generality or utility. It is to be expected, however, that their availability will lead to publications on their methodology which will rectify this situation. Some of these are APEX-3D,[239,240] PRO_LIGAND,[66,241] CATALYST,[242,243] and the suite of programs being developed at the University of Tokyo.[244,245]

LINKAGE WITH ANCILLARY METHODS FOR COMPUTATIONAL DRUG DESIGN

PHARMACOPHORE GENERATION

As can be seen from the above, 3D-QSAR has important contributions to make to other rapidly evolving areas of computational drug design. Increasingly, these methods, in spite of their only partially developed state, are being integrated into pharmacophore generation, database searching, de novo molecular design and combinatorial diversity software suites. How all this fits together in a practical setting is illustrated by Martin et al.[246] Automated pharmacophore generation methods such as DISCO[258] and others mentioned above[247] are proving invaluable in rapidly providing trial alignments for CoMFA. Other intriguing novel approaches have been described recently.[248-251]

DATABASE APPLICATIONS

The possibility of using CoMFA maps to screen databases is an attractive possibility which has been discussed by Clark et al[252] and implemented by Martin.[246] Indeed, most 3D-searching programs incorporate a shape-similarity evaluation for scoring or ranking hits.[253-256]

DE NOVO DESIGN

Lin and Martin described an interesting application of CoMFA to compare the diversity of new molecule sets designed either by chemists or by a de novo computer method.[257] CoMFA was used to show the greater diversity of the computer designed set as measured by a number of statistical methods. The new Tripos de novo design module, LEAPFROG,[19] includes the possibility of incorporating CoMFA fields into the search or screening strategy.

PROSPECTS

As can be seen from the above, the enormous amount of work reported on approaches to 3D-QSAR attests to the high interest in making these methods work. Good progress has been made in investigating some of the deficiencies with the original CoMFA procedure and creative alternatives and modifications have appeared which promise further progress with this method specifically. Furthermore, interesting alternative strategies have been demonstrated. It is worthwhile, however, to remind enthusiastic new users of these methods that care must be taken in applying and interpreting the methods and results. Behind the 3D is still QSAR, and all of the cautions which were raised when this promising and useful technique was first introduced still apply. This is especially true for those using the commercial implementation of CoMFA where it is possible to simply apply all program defaults and obtain what are characterized as "acceptable" or "predictive" models based on the "rules-of thumb" for statistical parameters Q^2, R^2 or s_{cv}. It should be clear from the above review that it is nearly always necessary to examine the effect of changing at least some of the program options, depending on the problem, to assess model stability, or indeed, even to detect a correlation in the first place. No default set of options can be accepted for all cases; those provided must only be used as a starting point. Grid size, scaling, positioning within the lattice, number of cross-validation groups, minimum sigma criterion: all have been shown in particular cases to have marked influence on the result. The statistical methods behind the analysis, while powerful and appropriate for the problem, are, nonetheless, very sophisticated, and, while good progress has been made in finding ways to use these in ways which assure that the models obtained are statistically robust, and even optimal, they in no way assure that the results obtained are meaningful in any physicochemical sense. Latent variables, while extracting the common information in the data set efficiently, can often hide distributional problems in the raw data that can lead to skewed or misleading results. In MLR, these problems are much easier to detect. With few exceptions, the composition and contribution of the latent variables have not been examined in CoMFA analyses. The work of Davis[64,65] and the GOLPE group[108] are notable exceptions, and show the value, if not the necessity of this. Other properties of PLS from a statistical viewpoint have been discussed by others.[105]

The many discussions and experiments to assess the adequacy of the parameters used in these methods underline increasingly how simple an approximation they give of the complexities of intermolecular interactions. For example, it now seems quite well established that hydrophobicity is not well approximated by the default CoMFA steric and electrostatic fields in the general case. Use of a water probe or a lipophilicity potential to generate a hydrophobicity field seems now to be desirable. Both of these expedients have been shown to capture this aspect of the binding interaction. Ironically, the most important insight of Hansch and Fujita in founding QSAR, that of the importance of lipophilicity, has had to be "rediscovered" to make 3D-QSAR work in many cases! Yet to be established is whether this additional field will be able to incorporate all of the entropic and solvation effects generally conceded to be important for binding. The steric and electrostatic fields appear to describe the enthalpic component of binding. There has been little examination so far of the behavior of CoMFA-like methods in situations where detailed thermodynamic information is available. The paper of Klebe et al[91] is pioneering in this regard.

From the perspective of traditional QSAR, the promise of CoMFA and other 3D methods has always been to provide an adequate description of steric effects, to better isolate regional intermolecular effects, electronic or steric, and to allow noncongeneric molecules to be included in the same analysis. How well have these methods lived up to these expectations? With regard to steric effects and shape, the record seems fairly promising. The predominant term in many CoMFA analyses has turned out to be the steric one, even when the field scaling is properly handled or when three probe types rather than two have been examined. The work of Martin et al on dopamine ligands is particularly notable,[163] and the same trend is seen in other studies of receptor ligand binding, e.g., GPCR ligands collected above. With regard to regional electronic effects, the record is still not clear. Electrostatic contributions to existing correlations are in many cases minor. In some cases these may be partial compensation for H-bonding effects that are missing due to lack of a hydrophobicity term. In others, the polar groups are an essential part of the pharmacophore and are hence present in all or most molecules. The variance of such features is thus low or nonexistent. No really good example of a CoMFA of bioisosteres has been reported where differences in the strength of the polar interaction are known to be the major determinant of activity. Examination of the contributions of the various latent variables to the CoMFA model might well provide more useful information on these cases. Finally, with regard to combining noncongeneric molecules in the same data set, the results, in my opinion, are still disappointing. Much of this may be due to the increasing realization that the alignment problem is still the key confounding feature of CoMFA and is, in the absence of receptor structure, a very arbitrary matter for noncongeneric series. The existence of multiple binding modes is turning out to be much more common and unpredictable than previously assumed.[146] The care that has been needed to obtain consistent CoMFAs, even when the bound complexes are available, shows that the derivation of a reliable CoMFA model is not a straightforward matter. Differential partitioning of binding energy between enthalpic and entropic effects for molecules acting at a common or overlapping binding site are nonadditive elements that can confound a CoMFA analysis.

CoMFA, in principle, is appropriate for analyzing interactions at the molecular level. The fields are used as parameters for specific intermolecular interactions. CoMFAs performed on biological data of a more complex nature, such as in vivo or toxicological potency seem very problematic from an interpretive standpoint, especially when compounds of mixed chemical type are included. It seems that in these cases, where lipophilicity has been established over the years to play such an important role, traditional Hansch analysis should be examined first. If successful, there is little to be gained by recasting this in CoMFA terms. A CoMFA may lead easily to spurious interpretations of apparent regional steric or electronic preferences. It is even hard to know how to interpret the very good correlation of Hammett σ values with CoMFA electrostatic fields. In physicochemical terms, the origin of these is presently hypothesized to be a combination of inductive electronic transmission through the molecular framework, polarization of π or σ electron structure and field transmission though space. The CoMFA field contours obtained in these correlations surround the substituents in regions distant from the affected carboxyl group in the benzoic acid study in a way that does not accord with chemical sensibility. Furthermore, of the three types of σ value, σ itself gives a better CoMFA than either σ_I (which might be expected to be better, being a field effect) or σ_R individually. This also does not make good chemical sense. It is notable that most of the studies applying CoMFA to generate traditional parameters of the principal property sort have concluded that these are probably not preferable to those derived in the traditional way.[90,125] When CoMFA analyses reproduce a traditional Hansch analysis, it should not be assumed that new information is being added due to the regional distribution of the CoMFA field distributions. CoMFA will necessarily partition global properties into regional contributions.

These comments are not meant to devalue in any way the work that has been done, but mainly to emphasize that 3D-QSAR is still very much an evolving technology. It is by no means a routine method for the casual user. We have much to learn about the proper use of the existing methodology and much to understand about what is still missing from an adequate description of binding energy estimation and correlation. New and creative approaches to these issues are appearing regularly now in the literature. There is no doubt that, in expanding its dimensions by one from 2D to 3D, QSAR has expanded its horizons by many fold and moved once more into the forefront of molecular design research.

REFERENCES

1. Hansch C, Fujita T. Pi-sigma-rho analysis. A method for the correlation of biological activity and chemical structure. J Am Chem Soc 1964; 86:1616-26.
2. Free SM, Jr, Wilson JW. A mathematical contribution to structure-activity studies. J Med Chem 1964; 7:395-9.
3. Kubinyi H. QSAR: Hansch Analysis and Related Approaches. Weinheim: VCH, 1994.
4. Fujita T. The extrathermodynamic approach to drug design. In: Ramsden CA, ed. Quantitative Drug Design. Oxford: Pergamon Press, 1990:497-560. (Hansch C, Sammes PG, Taylor JB, eds. Comprehensive Medicinal Chemistry; vol 4).
5. Hansch C, Leo A, Hoekman D. Exploring QSAR. Washington, DC: American Chemical Society, 1995.
6. Blaney JM, Hansch C. Application of molecular graphics to the analysis of macromolecular structures. In: Ramsden CA, ed. Quantitative Drug Design. Oxford: Pergamon, 1990:459-96. (Hansch C, Sammes PG, Taylor JB, eds. Comprehensive Medicinal Chemistry; vol 4).
7. C-QSAR. 3.55. BioByte Corp. Claremont, CA.
8. Kubinyi H. The Free-Wilson method and its relationship to the extrathermodynamic approach. In: Ramsden CA, ed. Quantitative Drug Design. Oxford: Pergamon, 1990:589-644. (Hansch C, Sammes PG, Taylor JB, eds. Comprehensive Medicinal Chemistry; vol 4).
9. Verloop A, Hoogenstraaten W, Tipker J. Development and application of new steric substituent parameters in drug design. In: Ariens EJ, ed. Drug Design. New York: Academic Press, 1976:165-207. vol 7.
10. Charton M. The quantitative description of steric effects. In: Zalewski RI, Krygowski TM, Shorter J, eds. Similarity Models in Organic Chemistry, Biochemistry and Related Fields. Amsterdam: Elsevier Science Publishers, 1991:629-87. Studies in Organic Chemistry; vol 42.
11. Silipo C, Vittoria A. Three-dimensional structure of drugs. In: Ramsden CA, ed. Quantitative Drug Design. Oxford: Pergamon, 1990:153-204. (Hansch C, Sammes PG, Taylor JB, eds. Comprehensive Medicinal Chemistry; vol 4).

12. Kato J, Ito MM, Tsuyuki M et al. A novel parameter (S1) for three-dimensional shape similarity between groups: correlation with molecular recognition and biological activity. J Chem Soc, Perkin Trans 1991; 2:131-6.

13. Randic M, Jerman-Blazic B, Trinajstic N. Development of 3-dimensional molecular descriptors. Comput Chem 1990; 14:237-46.

14. Hemkin HG, Lehmann PA. The use of computerized molecular structure scanning and principal component analysis to calculate molecular descriptors for QSAR. Quant Struct-Act Relat 1992; 11:332-8.

15. Hansch C, Sammes PG, Taylor JB, eds. Comprehensive Medicinal Chemistry. Oxford: Pergamon, 1990.

16. Kubinyi H, ed. 3D QSAR in Drug Design: Theory Methods and Applications. Leiden: ESCOM, 1993.

17. Cramer RD, III, Bunce JD. The DYLOMMS method: initial results from a comparative study of approaches to 3D QSAR. In: Hadzi D, Jerman-Blazic B, eds. QSAR in Drug Design and Toxicology. Amsterdam: Elsevier Science Publishers, 1987:3-12.

18. Cramer RD, III, Patterson DE, Bunce JD. Comparative molecular field analysis (CoMFA). 1. Effect of shape on binding of steroids to carrier proteins. J Am Chem Soc 1988; 110:5959-67.

19. SYBYL Molecular Modeling System. Tripos Assoc. St. Louis, MO.

20. Cramer RD, III, DePriest SA, Patterson DE et al. The developing practice of comparative molecular field analysis. In: Kubinyi H, ed. 3D QSAR in Drug Design: Theory Methods and Applications. Leiden: ESCOM, 1993:443-85.

21. Marshall GM, Naylor CB. Use of molecular graphics for structural analysis of small molecules. In: Ramsden CA, ed. Quantitative Drug Design. Oxford: Pergamon, 1990:431-58. (Hansch C, Sammes PG, Taylor JB, eds. Comprehensive Medicinal Chemistry; vol 4).

22. Marshall GM. Binding-site modeling of unknown receptors. In: Kubinyi H, ed. 3D QSAR in Drug Design: Theory Methods and Applications. Leiden: ESCOM, 1993:80-116.

23. Selassie CD, Klein TE. Building bridges: QSAR and molecular graphics. In: Kubinyi H, ed. 3D QSAR in Drug Design: Theory Methods and Applications. Leiden: ESCOM, 1993:257-75.

24. Simon Z. MTD and hyperstructure approaches. In: Kubinyi H, ed. 3D QSAR in Drug Design: Theory Methods and Applications. Leiden: ESCOM, 1993:307-19.

25. Burke BJ, Hopfinger AJ. Advances in molecular shape analysis. In: Kubinyi H, ed. 3D QSAR in Drug Design: Theory Methods and Applications. Leiden: ESCOM, 1993:276-306.

26. Ghose AK, Crippen GM. The distance geometry approach to modeling receptor sites. In: Ramsden CA, ed. Quantitative Drug Design. Oxford: Pergamon, 1990:715-34. vol 4.

27. Srivastava S, Richardson WW, Bradley MP et al. Three-dimensional receptor modeling using distance geometry and Voronoi polyhedra. In: Kubinyi H, ed. 3D QSAR in Drug Design: Theory Methods and Applications. Leiden: ESCOM, 1993:409-30.

28. Topliss JG, Costello RJ. Chance correlations in structure-activity studies using multiple regression analysis. J Med Chem 1972; 15:1066-8.

29. Topliss JG, Edwards RP. Chance factors in studies of quantitative structure-activity relationships. J Med Chem 1979; 22:1238-44.

30. Ciubotariu D, Deretey E, Oprea TI et al. Multiconformational minimal steric difference. Structure-acetylcholinesterase hydrolysis rates relations for acetic acid esters. Quant Struct Act Relat 1993; 12:367-72.

31. Oprea TI, Sulea TI, Ciubotariu D et al. QSAR by MTD for inhibition of keratinization of tracheal cells in organ culture by retinoids. In: Wermuth C-G, ed. Trends in QSAR and Molecular Modelling 92. Leiden: ESCOM, 1993:568-9.

32. Oprea TI, Ciubotariu D, Sulea TI et al. Comparison of the minimal steric difference (MTD) and comparative molecular field analysis (CoMFA) methods for analysis of binding of steroids to carrier proteins. Quant Struct Act Relat 1993; 12:21-6.

33. Hopfinger AJ, Burke BJ. Molecular shape analysis: a formalism to quantitatively establish spatial molecular similarity. In: Johnson MA, Maggiora GM, eds. Concepts in Applied Molecular Similarity. New York: Wiley, 1990:173-209.

34. Burke BJ, Dunn III WJ. Construction of a molecular shape analysis: three-dimensional quantitative structure-activity relationship for an analog series of pyridobenzodiazepinone inhibitors of muscarinic 2 and 3 receptors. J Med Chem 1994; 37:3775-88.

35. Tokarski JS, Hopfinger AJ. Three-dimensional molecular shape analysis-quantitative structure-activity relationship of a series of cholecystokinin-A receptor antagonists. J Med Chem 1994; 37:3639-54.

36. Rhyu KB, Patel HC, Hopfinger AJ. A 3D-QSAR study of anticoccidial triazines using molecular shape analysis. J Chem Inf Comput Sci 1995; 35:771-8.

37. Hopfinger AJ, Burke BJ, Dunn WJ, III. A generalized formalism of three-dimensional quantitative structure-property relationship analysis for flexible molecules using tensor representation. J Med Chem 1994; 37:3768-74.

38. Ghose AK, Crippen GM. Modeling the benzodiazepine receptor binding site by the general three-dimensional structure-directed quantitative structure-activity relationship method REMOTEDISC. Mol Pharmacol 1990; 37(5):725-34.

39. Ghose AK, Crippen GM, Revankar GR et al. Analysis of the in vitro antiviral activity of certain ribonucleosides against parainfluenza virus using a novel computer aided receptor modeling procedure. J Med Chem 1989; 32:746-56.

40. Viswanadhan VN, Ghose AK, Weinstein JN. Mapping the binding site of the nucleoside transporter protein: a 3D-QSAR study. Biochim Biophys Acta 1990; 1039:356-66.

41. Ghose AK, Logan ME, Treasurywala AM et al. Determination of pharmacophoric geometry for collagenase inhibitors using a novel computational method and its verification using molecular dynamics, NMR, and X-ray crystallography. J Am Chem Soc 1995; 117:4671-82.

42. Donne-Op den Kelder GM, Bultsma T, Timmerman H et al. Mapping of the β2-adrenergic receptor on Chang liver cells. Differences between high- and low-affinity receptor states. J Med Chem 1988; 31:1060-79.

43. Linschoten MR, Bultsma T, IJzerman AP et al. Mapping the turkey erythrocyte beta receptor: a distance geometry approach. J Med Chem 1986; 29:278-86.

44. Crippen GM. Voronoi binding site models. J Comput Chem 1987; 8:943-55.

45. Crippen GM, Bradley MP, Richardson WW. Why are binding-site models more complicated than molecules? Perspect Drug Discovery Des 1993; 1:321-8.

46. Srivastava S, Crippen GM. Analysis of cocaine receptor site ligand binding by three-dimensional Voronoi site modeling approach. J Med Chem 1993; 36:3572-9.

47. Bradley M, Richardson W, Crippen GM. Deducing molecular similarity using Voronoi binding sites. J Chem Inf Comput Sci 1993; 33:750-5.

48. Bradley MP, Crippen GM. Voronoi modeling: the binding of triazines and pyrimidines to L. casei dihydrofolate reductase. J Med Chem 1993; 36:3171-7.

49. Carroll FI, Gao Y, Rahman MA et al. Synthesis, ligand binding, QSAR, and CoMFA study of 3β-(p-substituted phenyl)tropane-2β-carboxylic acid methyl esters. J Med Chem 1991; 34:2719-25.

50. Crippen G. Intervals and the deduction of drug binding site models. J Comp Chem 1995; 16:486-500.

51. Wade RC. Molecular interaction fields. In: Kubinyi H, ed. 3D QSAR in Drug Design: Theory Methods and Applications. Leiden: ESCOM, 1993:486-505.

52. Politzer P, Murray JS. Chemical applications of molecular electrostatic potentials. Trans Am Crystallogr Assoc 1993; 26:23-39.

53. Abraham DJ, Kellogg GE. Hydrophobic fields. In: Kubinyi H, ed. 3D QSAR in Drug Design: Theory Methods and Applications. Leiden: ESCOM, 1993:506-22.

54. Finn PW. The calculation, representation and analysis of molecular fields. In: Vinter JG, Gardener M, eds. Molecular Modelling and Drug Design. Boca Raton: CRC Press, 1994:266-304.

55. Naray-Szabo G. Analysis of molecular recognition: steric, electrostatic and hydrophobic complementarity. J Molec Recogn 1993; 6:205-10.

56. Wold S, Johansson E, Cocchi M. PLS—partial least-squares projections to latent structures. In: Kubinyi H, ed. 3D QSAR in Drug Design: Theory Methods and Applications. Leiden: ESCOM, 1993:523-50.

57. Thibaut U. Applications of CoMFA and related 3D QSAR approaches. In: Kubinyi H, ed. 3D QSAR in Drug Design: Theory Methods and Applications. Leiden: ESCOM, 1993:661-96.

58. Wade RC, Clark KJ, Goodford PJ. Further development of hydrogen bond functions for use in determining energetically favorable binding sites on molecules of known structure. 1. Ligand probe groups with the ability to form two hydrogen bonds. J Med Chem 1993; 36:140-7.

59. Wade RC, Goodford PJ. Further development of hydrogen bond functions for use in determining energetically favorable binding sites on molecules of known structure. 2. Ligand probe groups with the ability to form more than two hydrogen bonds. J Med Chem 1993; 36:148-56.

60. Goodford PJ. A computational procedure for determining energetically favorable binding sites on biologically important macromolecules. J Med Chem 1985; 28:849-57.

61. Boobbyer DNA, Goodford PJ, McWhinnie PM et al. New hydrogen-bond potentials for use in determining energetically favorable binding sites on molecules of known structure. J Med Chem 1989; 32:1083-94.

62. Kim KH, Martin YC. Direct prediction of linear free energy substituent effects from 3D structures using comparative molecular field analysis. 1. Electronic effects of substituted benzoic acids. J Org Chem 1991; 56:2723-9.

63. Norinder U. Theoretical amino acid descriptors. Application to bradykinin potentiating peptides. Peptides 1991; 12:1223-7.

64. Davis AM, Gensmantel NP, Johansson E et al. The use of the GRID program in the 3-D QSAR analysis of a series of calcium-channel agonists. J Med Chem 1994; 37:963-72.

65. Davis AM. 3D QSAR methods. In: van de Waterbeemd H, ed. Advanced Computer-Assisted Techniques in Drug Discovery.

Weinheim: VCH, 1995:39-60. (Mannhold R, Krogsgaard-Larsen P, Timmerman H, eds. Methods and Principals of Medicinal Chemistry; vol 3).

66. Waszkowycz B, Clark DE, Frenkel D et al. PRO_LIGAND: An approach to de novo molecular design. 2. Design of novel molecules from molecular field analysis (MFA) models and pharmacophores. J Med Chem 1994; 37:3994-4002.

67. Gasteiger J, Marsili M. Iterative partial equalization of orbital electronegativity—a rapid access to atomic charges. Tetrahedron 1980; 36:3219-28.

68. Kellogg GE, Joshi GS, Abraham DJ. New tools for modeling and understanding hydrophobicity and hydrophobic interactions. Med Chem Res 1991; 1:444-53.

69. Kellogg GE, Semus SF, Abraham DJ. HINT: a new method of empirical hydrophobic field calculation for CoMFA. J Comput Aided Mol Des 1991; 5:545-52.

70. Cruciani G, Watson KA. Comparative molecular field analysis using GRID force-field and GOLPE variable selection methods in a study of inhibitors of glycogen phosphorylase b. J Med Chem 1994; 37:2589-601.

71. Cocchi M, Cruciani G, Menziani MC et al. Use of advanced chemometric tools and comparison of different 3D descriptors in QSAR analysis of prazosin analog α1-adrenergic antagonists. In: Wermuth C-G, ed. Trends in QSAR and Molecular Modelling 92. Leiden: ESCOM, 1993:527-9.

72. Cocchi M, Johansson E. Amino acid characterization by GRID and multivariate data analysis. Quant Struct-Act Relat 1993; 12:1-8.

73. Kim KH, Greco G, Novellino E et al. Use of the hydrogen bond potential function in a comparative molecular field analysis (CoMFA) on a set of benzodiazepines. J Comput Aided Mol Des 1993; 7:263-80.

74. GRID. 12. Molecular Discovery, Ltd. Oxford.

75. HINT. 2.0. eduSoft, LC. Ashland, VA.

76. Gaillard P, Carrupt PA, Testa B et al. Molecular lipophilicity potential, a tool in 3D QSAR: method and applications. J Comput-Aided Mol Des 1994; 8:83-96.

77. Kenny PW. Prediction of hydrogen bond basicity from computed molecular electrostatic properties: implications for comparative molecular field analysis. J Chem Soc, Perkin Trans 1994; 2:199-202.

78. Waller CL, Marshall GR. 3D-QSAR three-dimensional quantitative structure-activity relationship of angiotensin-converting enzyme and thermolysin inhibitors. II. A comparison of CoMFA models incorporating molecular orbital fields and desolvation free energies based on active-analog and complementary-receptor-field alignment rules. J Med Chem 1993; 36:2390-403.

79. Poso A, Tuppurainen K, Gynther J. Modeling of molecular mutagenicity with comparative molecular field analysis (CoMFA). Structural and electronic properties of MX compounds related to TA100 mutagenicity. Theochem 1994; 110:255-60.

80. Martin YC, Bures MG, Danaher EA et al. A fast new approach to pharmacophore mapping and its application to dopaminergic and benzodiazepine agonists. J Comput Aided Mol Des 1993; 7:83-102.

81. Dammkoehler RA, Karasek SF, Shands EFB et al. Constrained search of conformational hyperspace. J Comput Aided Mol Des 1989; 3:3-21.

82. Prendergast K, Adams K, Greenlee WJ et al. Derivation of a 3D pharmacophore model for the angiotensin-II site one receptor. J Comput-Aided Mol Des 1994; 8:491-512.

83. Klebe G, Abraham U, Mietzner T. Molecular similarity indices in a comparative analysis (CoMSIA) of drug molecules to correlate and predict their biological activity. J Med Chem 1994; 37:4130-46.

84. Kearsley SK, Smith GM. An alternate method for the alignment of molecular structures; maximizing electrostatic and steric overlap. Tetrahedron Comput Method 1990; 3:615-33.

85. Horwitz JP, Massova I, Wiese TE et al. Comparative molecular field analysis of in vitro growth inhibition of L1210 and HCT-8 cells by some pyrazoloacridines. J Med Chem 1993; 36:3511-16.

86. Horwitz JP, Massova I, Wiese TE et al. Comparative molecular field analysis of the antitumor activity of 9H-thioxanthen-9-one derivatives against pancreatic ductal carcinoma 03. J Med Chem 1994; 37:781-6.

87. Klebe G, Mietzner T, Weber F. Different approaches toward an automatic structural alignment of drug molecules: applications to sterol mimics, thrombin and thermolysin inhibitors. J Comput Aided Mol Des 1994; 8:751-78.

88. Calder JA, Wyatt JA, Frenkel DA et al. CoMFA validation of the superposition of six classes of compounds which block GABA receptors noncompetitively. J Comput Aided Mol Des 1993; 7:45-60.

89. Folkers G, Merz A, Rognan D. CoMFA: scope and limitations. In: Kubinyi H, ed. 3D QSAR in Drug Design: Theory Methods and Applications. Leiden: ESCOM, 1993:583-618.

90. van de Waterbeemd H, Clementi S, Costantino G et al. CoMFA-derived substituent descriptors for structure-property correlations. In: Kubinyi H, ed. 3D QSAR in Drug Design: Theory Methods and Applications. Leiden: ESCOM, 1993:697-707.

91. Klebe G, Abraham U. On the prediction of binding properties of drug molecules by comparative molecular field analysis. J Med Chem 1993; 36:70-80.

92. Raghavan K, Buolamwini JK, Fesen MR et al. Three-dimensional quantitative structure-activity relationship (QSAR) of HIV integrase

inhibitors: a comparative molecular field analysis (CoMFA) study. J Med Chem 1995; 38:890-7.

93. van Steen BJ, van Wijngaarden I, Tulp MTM et al. Structure-affinity relationship studies on 5-HT1A receptor ligands. 2. Heterobicyclic phenylpiperazines with N4-aralkyl substituents. J Med Chem 1994; 37:2761-73.

94. Kim KH. Use of the hydrogen-bond potential function in comparative molecular field analysis (CoMFA): An extension of CoMFA. In: Wermuth C-G, ed. Trends in QSAR and Molecular Modelling 92. Leiden: ESCOM, 1993:245-51.

95. Nayak VR, Kellogg GE. Cyclodextrin-barbiturate inclusion complexes: A CoMFA/HINT 3-D QSAR study. Med Chem Res 1994; 3:491-502.

96. Oprea TI, Waller CL, Marshall GR. 3D-QSAR of human immunodeficiency virus (I) protease inhibitors. III. Interpretation of CoMFA results. Drug Design Discovery 1994; 12:29-51.

97. Waller CL. A three-dimensional technique for the calculation of octanol-water partition coefficients. Quant Struct Act Relat 1994; 13:172-6.

98. DePriest SA, Mayer D, Naylor CB et al. 3D-QSAR of angiotensin-converting enzyme and thermolysin inhibitors: a comparison of CoMFA models based on deduced and experimentally determined active site geometries. J Am Chem Soc 1993; 115:5372-84.

99. Greco G, Novellino E, Pellecchia M et al. Effects of variable selection on CoMFA coefficient contour maps in a set of triazines inhibiting DHFR. J Comput Aided Mol Des 1994; 8:97-112.

100. Kim KH. Use of indicator variable in comparative molecular field analysis. Med Chem Res 1993; 3:257-67.

101. Kroemer RT, Hecht P. Replacement of steric 6-12 potential-derived interaction energies by atom-based indicator variables in CoMFA leads to models of higher consistency. J Comput-Aided Mol Des 1995; 9:205-12.

102. Waller CL, Oprea TI, Giolitti A et al. Three-dimensional QSAR of human immunodeficiency virus (I) protease inhibitors. 1. A CoMFA study employing experimentally-determined alignment rules. J Med Chem 1993; 36:4152-60.

103. Oprea TI, Waller CL, Marshall GR. Three-dimensional quantitative structure-activity relationship of human immunodeficiency virus (I) protease inhibitors. 2. Predictive power using limited exploration of alternate binding modes. J Med Chem 1994; 37:2206-15.

104. Cramer RD, III. Partial least squares (PLS): its strengths and limitations. Perspect Drug Discovery Des 1993; 1:269-78.

105. Kubinyi H, Abraham U. Practical problems in PLS analyses. In: Kubinyi H, ed. 3D QSAR in Drug Design: Theory Methods and Applications. Leiden: ESCOM, 1993:717-28.

106. Baroni M, Costantino G, Cruciani G et al. GOLPE: an advanced chemometric tool for 3D QSAR problems. In: Wermuth C-G, ed. Trends in QSAR and Molecular Modelling 92. Leiden: ESCOM, 1993:256-9.

107. Baroni M, Costantino G, Cruciani G et al. Generating optimal linear PLS estimations (GOLPE): an advanced chemometric tool of handling 3D-QSAR problems. Quant Struct Act Relat 1993; 12:9-20.

108. Cruciani G, Clementi S. GOLPE: philosophy and applications in 3D QSAR. In: van de Waterbeemd H, ed. Advanced Computer-Assisted Techniques in Drug Discovery. Weinheim: VCH, 1995:61-88. (Mannhold R, Krogsgaard-Larsen P, Timmerman H, eds. Methods and Principals of Medicinal Chemistry; vol 3).

109. Norinder U. Experimental design based 3-D QSAR analysis of steroid-protein interactions: application to human CBG complexes. J Comput Aided Mol Des 1990; 4:381-9.

110. Cho SJ, Tropsha A. Cross-validated R2-guided region selection for comparative molecular field analysis: a simple method to achieve consistent results. J Med Chem 1995; 38:1060-6.

111. Caliendo G, Greco G, Novellino E et al. Combined use of factorial design and comparative molecular field analysis (CoMFA): a case study. Quant Struct-Act Relat 1994; 13:249-61.

112. Novellino E, Fattorusso C, Greco G. Use of comparative field analysis and cluster analysis in series design. Pharmaceutica Acta Helvetiae 1995; 70:149-54.

113. Bush BL, Nachbar RB, Jr. Sample-distance partial least squares: PLS optimized for many variables, with application to CoMFA. J Comput Aided Mol Des 1993; 7:587-619.

114. Martin YC, Lin CT, Hetti C et al. PLS analysis of distance matrixes to detect nonlinear relationships between biological potency and molecular properties. J Med Chem 1995; 38:3009-15.

115. Clementi S, Cruciani G, Riganelli D et al. Autocorrelation as a tool for a congruent description of molecules in 3D-QSAR studies. Pharm Pharmacol Lett 1993; 3:5-8.

116. Clementi S, Cruciani G, Baroni M et al. Series design. In: Kubinyi H, ed. 3D QSAR in Drug Design: Theory Methods and Applications. Leiden: ESCOM, 1993:567-82.

117. Krystek Jr, SR, Hunt JT, Stein PD et al. Three-dimensional quantitative structure-activity relationships of sulfonamide endothelin inhibitors. J Med Chem 1995; 38:659-68.

118. van de Waterbeemd H, Carrupt PA, Testa B et al. Multivariate data modeling of new steric, topological and CoMFA-derived substituent parameters. In: Wermuth C-G, ed. Trends in QSAR and Molecular Modelling 92. Leiden: ESCOM, 1993:69-75.

119. Hocart SJ, Reddy V, Murphy WA et al. Three-dimensional quantitative structure-activity relationships of somatostatin analogs. 1. Comparative molecular field analysis of growth hormone release-inhibiting potencies. J Med Chem 1995; 38:1974-89.

120. Debnath AK, Hansch C, Kim KH et al. Mechanistic interpretation of the genotoxicity of nitrofurans (antibacterial agents) using quantitative structure-activity relationships and comparative molecular field analysis. J Med Chem 1993; 36:1007-16.

121. Simon Z. Comparative molecular field analysis. Critical comments. Rev Roum Chim 1992; 37:323-5.

122. Carrieri A, Altomare C, Barreca ML et al. Papain catalyzed hydrolysis of aryl esters: a comparison of the Hansch, Docking and CoMFA methods. Farmaco, Ed Sci 1994; 49:573-85.

123. Kim KH. Comparison of classical and 3D QSAR. In: Kubinyi H, ed. 3D QSAR in Drug Design: Theory Methods and Applications. Leiden: ESCOM, 1993:619-42.

124. Carroll FI, Mascarella SW, Kuzemko MA et al. Synthesis, Ligand Binding, and QSAR (CoMFA and Classical) Study of 3β-(3'-Substituted phenyl)-, 3β-(4'-Substituted phenyl)-, and 3β-(3',4'-Disubstituted phenyl)tropane-2β-carboxylic Acid Methyl Esters. J Med Chem 1994; 37:2865-73.

125. Norinder U. A PLS QSAR analysis using 3D generated aromatic descriptors of principal property type: application to some dopamine D2 benzamide antagonists. J Comput Aided Mol Des 1993; 7:671-82.

126. Norinder U, Jonsson J. Theoretical descriptors of nucleic acid bases. Application to DNA promoter sequences. Quant Struct-Act Relat 1994; 13:295-301.

127. Langer T. Molecular similarity determination of heteroaromatics using CoMFA and multivariate data analysis. Quant Struct-Act Relat 1994; 13:402-5.

128. Good AC, So SS, Richards WG. Structure-activity relationships from molecular similarity matrices. J Med Chem 1993; 36:433-8.

129. Jain AN, Koile K, Chapman D. Compass: Predicting Biological Activities from Molecular Surface Properties. Performance Comparisons on a Steroid Benchmark. J Med Chem 1994; 37:2315-27.

130. Norinder U. 3-D QSAR analysis of steroid/protein interactions: the use of difference maps. J Comput Aided Mol Des 1991; 5:419-26.

131. Rum G, Herndon WC. Molecular similarity concepts. 5. Analysis of steroid-protein binding constants. J Am Chem Soc 1991; 113:9055-60.

132. Good AC, Peterson SJ, Richards WG. QSAR's from similarity matrices. Technique validation and application in the comparison of different similarity evaluation methods. J Med Chem 1993; 36:2929-37.

133. Hahn M, Rogers D. Receptor surface models. 2. Application to quantitative structure-activity relationships studies. J Med Chem 1995; 38:2091-102.

134. Wagener M, Sadowski J, Gasteiger J. Autocorrelation of Molecular Surface Properties for Modeling Corticosteroid Binding Globulin and Cytosolic Ah Receptor Activity by Neural Networks. J Am Chem Soc 1995; 117:7769-75.

135. Clementi S. Statistics and drug design. In: Jolles G, Wooldridge KRH, eds. Drug Design: Fact or Fantasy? New York: Academic Press, 1984.

136. Allen MS, LaLoggia AJ, Dorn LJ et al. Predictive binding of β-ONB-carboline inverse agonists and antagonists via the CoMFA/GOLPE approach. J Med Chem 1992; 35:4001-10.

137. DePriest SA, Shands EFB, Dammkoehler RA et al. 3D-QSAR: further studies on inhibitors of angiotensin-converting enzyme. Pharmacochem Libr 1991; 16:405-14.

138. Motoc I, Dammkoehler RA, Mayer D et al. Three-dimensional quantitative structure-activity relationships. I. General approach to the pharmacophore model validation. Quant Struct Act Relat 1986; 5:99-105.

139. Hansch C. Quantitative structure-activity relationships and the unnamed science. Acc Chem Res 1993; 26:147-53.

140. Altomare C, Campagna F, Carta V et al. Synthesis, benzodiazepine receptor affinity and anticonvulsant activity of 5-H-indeno [1,2-c]pyridazine derivatives. Farmaco 1994; 49:313-23.

141. Greco G, Novellino E, Fiorini I et al. A comparative molecular field analysis model for 6-arylpyrrolo[2,1-d][1,5]benzothiazepines binding selectively to the mitochondrial benzodiazepine receptor. J Med Chem 1994; 37:4100-8.

142. Wong G, Koehler KF, Skolnick P et al. Synthetic and computer-assisted analysis of the structural requirements for selective, high-affinity ligand binding to diazepam-insensitive benzodiazepine receptors. J Med Chem 1993; 36:1820-30.

143. Crippen GM. Distance geometry analysis of the benzodiazepine binding site. Mol Pharmacol 1982; 22:11-9.

144. Hadjipavlou-Litina D, Hansch C. Quantitative structure-activity relationships of the benzodiazepines. A review and reevaluation. Chem Rev 1994; 94:1483-505.

145. Zhang W, Koehler KF, Zhang P et al. Development of a comprehensive pharmacophore model for the benzodiazepine receptor. Drug Design Discovery 1995; 12:193-248.

146. Mattos C, Ringe D. Multiple binding modes. In: Kubinyi H, ed. 3D QSAR in Drug Design: Theory Methods and Applications. Leiden: ESCOM, 1993:226-56.

147. Badger J, Minor I, Oliviera MA et al. Structural analysis of antiviral agents that interact with the capsid of human rhinoviruses. Protein Struct Funct Genetics 1989; 6:1-19.

148. Diana GD, Nitz TJ, Mallamo JP et al. Antipicornavirus compounds: use of rational drug design and molecular modelling. Antiviral Chem Chemother 1993; 4:1-10.

149. Diana GD, Kowalczyk P, Treasurywala AM et al. CoMFA analysis of the interactions of antipicornavirus compounds in the binding pocket of human rhinovirus-14. J Med Chem 1992; 35:1002-8.

150. Diana GD, Kowalczyk P, Treasurywala AM et al. CoMFA analysis of the interactions of antipicornavirus compounds in the binding pocket of human rhinovirus-14. J Med Chem 1992; 35:1002-8.

151. Thibaut U, Folkers G, Klebe G et al. Editorial. Recommendations for CoMFA studies and 3D QSAR publications. Quant Struct-Act Relat 1994; 13:1-3.

152. Thibaut U, Folkers G, Klebe G et al. Appendix A. Recommendations for CoMFA studies and 3D QSAR publications. In: Kubinyi H, ed. 3D QSAR in Drug Design: Theory Methods and Applications. Leiden: ESCOM, 1993:711-6.

153. Leo A. Hydrophobic parameter: measurement and calculation. In: Methods in Enzymology. New York: Academic Press, 1991; 202:544-55.

154. Kim KH. 3D-quantitative structure-activity relationships: describing hydrophobic interactions directly from 3D structures using a comparative molecular field analysis (CoMFA) approach. Quant Struct Act Relat 1993; 12:232-8.

155. Kim KH. Description of the reversed-phase high-performance liquid chromatography (RP-HPLC) capacity factors and octanol-water partition coefficients of 2-pyrazine and 2-pyridine analogues directly from the three-dimensional structures using comparative molecular field analysis (CoMFA) approach. Quant Struct Act Relat 1995; 14:8-18.

156. Kim KH. 3D-Quantitative structure-activity relationships: description of electronic effects directly from 3D structures using a GRID-comparative molecular field analysis (CoMFA) approach. Quant Struct Act Relat 1992; 11:127-34.

157. Kim KH, Martin YC. Evaluation of electrostatic and steric descriptors for 3D-QSAR: The hydrogen ion and methyl group probes using comparative molecular field analysis (CoMFA) and the modified partial least squares method. In: Silipo C, Vittoria A, eds. QSAR: Rational Approaches to the Design of Bioactive Compounds. Amsterdam: Elsevier Science Publishers, 1991:151-4.

158. Kim KH. 3D-Quantitative structure-activity relationships: investigation of steric effects with descriptors directly from 3D structures

using a comparative molecular field analysis (CoMFA) approach. Quant Struct Act Relat 1992; 11:453-60.

159. Charton M, Charton BI. The structural dependence of amino acid hydrophobicity parameters. J Theor Biol 1982; 99:629-44.

160. Steinmetz WE. A CoMFA analysis of selected physical properties of amino acids in water. Quant Struct Act Relat 1995; 14:19-23.

161. Kim KH, Martin YC. Direct prediction of dissociation constants (pKa's) of clonidine-like imidazolines, 2-substituted imidazoles and 1-methyl-2-substituted-imidazoles from 3D structures using a comparative molecular field analysis (CoMFA) approach. J Med Chem 1991; 34:2056-60.

162. Liu R, Matheson LE. Comparative molecular field analysis combined with physicochemical parameters for prediction of polydimethylsiloxane membrane flux in isopropanol. Pharm Res 1994; 11:257-66.

163. Martin YC, Lin CT, Wu J. Application of CoMFA to D1 dopaminergic agonists: a case study. In: Kubinyi H, ed. 3D QSAR in Drug Design. Leiden: ESCOM, 1993:643-60.

164. Minor DL, Wyrick SD, Charifson PS et al. Synthesis and molecular modeling of 1-phenyl-1,2,3,4-tetrahydroisoquinolines and related 5,6,8,9-tetrahydro-13bh-dibenzo[a,h]quinolizines as D1 dopamine antagonists. J Med Chem 1994; 37:4317-28.

165. Charifson PS, Bowen JP, Wyrick SD et al. Conformational analysis and molecular modeling of 1-phenyl-, 4-phenyl-, and 1-benzyl-1,2,3,4-tetrahydroisoquinolines as D1 dopamine receptor ligands. J Med Chem 1989; 32:2050-8.

166. Norinder U, Höegberg T. A quantitative structure-activity relationship for some dopamine D2 antagonists of benzamide type. Acta Pharm Nord 1992; 4:73-8.

167. Liegeois JF, Dupont L, Delarge J. Application of comparative molecular field analysis (CoMFA) to the study of heterocyclic analogs of clozapine. J Pharm Belg 1992; 47:100-8.

168. El-Bermawy MA, Lotter H, Glennon RA. Comparative molecular field analysis of the binding of arylpiperazines at 5-HT1A serotonin receptors. Med Chem Res 1992; 2:290-7.

169. Langlois M, Bremont B, Rousselle D et al. Structural analysis by the comparative molecular field analysis method of the affinity of β-adrenoreceptor blocking agents for 5-HT1A and 5-HT1B receptors. Eur J Pharmacol, Mol Pharmacol Sect 1993; 244:77-87.

170. Agarwal A, Taylor EW. 3-D QSAR for intrinsic activity of 5-HT1A receptor ligands by the method of comparative molecular field analysis. J Comput Chem 1993; 14:237-45.

171. Agarwal A, Pearson PP, Taylor EW et al. Three-dimensional quantitative structure-activity relationships of 5-HT receptor binding data

for tetrahydropyridinylindole derivatives: a comparison of the Hansch and CoMFA methods. J Med Chem 1993; 36:4006-14.

172. Taylor EW, Nikam SS, Lambert G et al. Molecular determinants for recognition of RU 24969 analogs at central 5-Hydroxytryptamine recognition sites: use of a bilinear function and substituent volumes to describe steric fit. Mol Pharmacol 1988; 34:42-53.

173. Greco G, Novellino E, Silipo C et al. Comparative molecular field analysis on a set of muscarinic agonists. Quant Struct Act Relat 1991; 10:289-99.

174. Bolognese A, Diurno MV, Greco G et al. Quantitative structure-activity relationships in a set of thiazolidin-4-ones acting as H1-histamine antagonists. J Recept Signal Transduction Res 1995; 15:631-41.

175. Rault S, Bureau R, Pilo JC et al. Comparative molecular field analysis of CCK-A antagonists using field-fit as an alignment technique. A convenient guide to design new CCK-A ligands. J Comput Aided Mol Des 1992; 6:553-68.

176. Bureau R, Rault S, Robba M. Comparative molecular field analysis of CCK-B antagonists. Eur J Med Chem 1994; 29:487-94.

177. Thomas BF, Compton DR, Martin BR et al. Modeling the cannabinoid receptor: a three-dimensional quantitative structure-activity analysis. Mol Pharmacol 1991; 40:656-65.

178. Ablordeppey SY, El-Ashmawy MB, Glennon RA. Analysis of the structure-activity relationships of sigma receptor ligands. Med Chem Res 1992; 1:425-38.

179. Myers AM, Charifson PS, Owens CE et al. Conformational analysis, pharmacophore identification, and comparative molecular field analysis of ligands for the neuromodulatory sigma3 receptor. J Med Chem 1994; 37:4109-17.

180. Mascarella SW, Bai X, Williams W et al. (+)-cis-N-(para-, meta-, and ortho-substituted benzyl)-N-normetazocines: Synthesis and binding affinity at the [3H]-(+)-pentazocine-labeled (sigma1) site and quantitative structure-affinity relationship studies. J Med Chem 1995; 38:565-9.

181. Allen MS, Tan YC, Trudell ML et al. Synthetic and computer-assisted analyses of the pharmacophore for the benzodiazepine receptor inverse agonist site. J Med Chem 1990; 33:2343-57.

182. Ohta M, Koga H, Sato H et al. Comparative molecular field analysis of benzopyran-4-carbothioamide potassium channel openers. Bioorg Med Chem Lett 1994; 4:2903-6.

183. Welch W, Ahmad S, Airey JA et al. Structural determinants of high-affinity binding of ryanoids to the vertebrate skeletal muscle ryanodine receptor: a comparative molecular field analysis. Biochemistry 1994; 33:6074-85.

184. Waller CL, Wyrick SD, Kemp WE et al. Conformational analysis, molecular modeling, and quantitative structure-activity relationship studies of agents for the inhibition of astrocytic chloride transport. Pharm Res 1994; 11:47-53.

185. Davis AM, Gensmantel NP, Marriott DP. Use of the GRID program in the 3D QSAR of a series of calcium channel agonists. In: Wermuth C-G, ed. Trends in QSAR and Molecular Modelling 92. Leiden: ESCOM, 1993:517-18.

186. SIMCA. 4.4. Umetri, A.B. Umea, Sweden.

187. Anzini M, Cappelli A, Vomero S et al. Novel, potent, and selective 5-HT3 receptor antagonists based on the arylpiperazine skeleton: Synthesis, structure, biological activity and comparative molecular field analysis studies. J Med Chem 1995; 38:2692-704.

188. Langer T, Wermuth CG. Inhibitors of prolyl endopeptidase: Characterization of the pharmacophoric pattern using conformational analysis and 3D-QSAR. J Comput Aided Mol Des 1993; 7:253-62.

189. Blankley CJ, White AD. Lipophilic and electronic factors influencing the activity of a series of urea ACAT inhibitors: approaches to model specification. In: Wermuth C-G, ed. Trends in QSAR and Molecular Modelling 92. Leiden: ESCOM, 1993:349-51.

190. Miyashita Y, Shiraishi Y, Hasegawa K et al. Partial least squares modelling of HMG CoA reductase inhibitors. In: Doyama M, Kihara J, Tanaka M, Yamamota R, eds. Computer Aided Innovation of New Materials. Amsterdam: Elsevier Sciences Publishers, 1993:vol 2.

191. Brandt W, Lehmann T, Willkomm C et al. CoMFA investigations of two series of artificial peptide inhibitors of serine protease thermitase. Int J Peptide Protein Res 1995; 46:73-8.

192. Altomare C, Carrupt P-A, Gaillard P et al. Quantitative structure-metabolism relationship analyses of MAO-mediated toxication of 1-methyl-4-phenyl-1,2,3,6-tetrahydropyridine and analogues. Chem Res Toxicol 1992; 5:366-75.

193. Carroll FI, Abraham P, Lewin AH et al. Pharmacophore development of (-)-cocaine analogs for the dopamine, serotonin, and norepinephrine uptake sites using a QSAR and CoMFA approach. In: Wermuth C-G, ed. Trends in QSAR and Molecular Modelling 92. Leiden: ESCOM, 1993:530-1.

194. Loughney DA, Schwender CF. A comparison of progestin and androgen receptor binding using the CoMFA technique. J Comput Aided Mol Des 1992; 6:569-81.

195. Gantchev TG, Ali H, van Lier JE. Quantitative structure-activity relationships/comparative molecular field analysis (QSAR/CoMFA) for Receptor-binding properties of halogenated estradiol derivatives. J Med Chem 1994; 37:4164-76.

196. Czaplinski K-HA, Grunewald GL. A comparative molecular field analysis derived model of the binding of Taxol analogs to microtubules. Bioorg Med Chem Lett 1994; 4:2211-16.

197. Debnath AK, Jiang S, Strick N et al. Three-dimensional structure-activity analysis of a series of porphyrin derivatives with anti-HIV-1 activity targeted to the V3 loop of the gp120 envelope glycoprotein of the human immunodeficiency virus type 1. J Med Chem 1994; 37:1099-108.

198. Avery MA, Gao F, Chong WKM et al. Structure-activity relationships of the antimalarial agent artemisinin. 1. Synthesis and comparative molecular field analysis of C-9 analogs of artemisinin and 10-deoxoartemisinin. J Med Chem 1993; 36:4264-75.

199. Harpalani AD, Snyder SW, Subramanyam B et al. Alkylamides as inducers of human leukemia cell differentiation: a quantitative structure-activity relationship study using comparative molecular field analysis. Cancer Res 1993; 53:766-71.

200. Akamatsu M, Nishimura K, Osabe H et al. Quantitative structure-activity studies of pyrethroids. 29. Comparative molecular field analysis (three-dimensional) of the knockdown activity of substituted benzyl chrysanthemates and tetramethrin and related imido- and lactam-N-carbinyl esters. Pestic Biochem Physiol 1994; 48:15-30.

201. Greco G, Novellino E, Pellecchia M et al. Use of the hydrophobic substituent constant in a comparative molecular field analysis (CoMFA) on a set of anilides inhibiting the Hill reaction. Sar Qsar Environ Res 1993; 1:301-34.

202. Briens F, Bureau R, Rault S et al. Comparative molecular field analysis of chlorophenols. Application in ecotoxicology. Sar Qsar Environ Res 1994; 2:147-57.

203. Johnson MA, Maggiora GM, eds. Concepts and Applications of Molecular Similarity. New York: John Wiley & Sons, 1990.

204. Johnson MA, Maggiora GM, Lajiness MS et al. Molecular similarity analysis: applications in drug discovery. In: van de Waterbeemd H, ed. Advanced Computer-Assisted Techniques in Drug Discovery. Weinheim: VCH, 1995:89-110. (Mannhold R, Krogsgaard-Larsen P, Timmerman H, eds. Methods and Principles of Medicinal Chemistry; vol 3).

205. Dean PM. Molecular similarity. In: Kubinyi H, ed. 3D QSAR in Drug Design: Theory Methods and Applications. Leiden: ESCOM, 1993:150-72.

206. Richards WG, Hodgkin EE. Molecular similarity. Chem Britain 1988; 24:1143-4.

207. Takahashi Y. Identification of structural similarity of organic molecules. Top Curr Chem 1995; 174:105-33.

208. Good AC. The calculation of molecular similarity: alternative formulas, data manipulation and graphical display. J Mol Graphics 1992; 10:144-51.

209. Csorvassy I, Tozser L, Karpati L et al. The molecular transform as a similarity measure. J Math Chem 1993; 13:343-57.

210. Ponec R, Strnad M. Position invariant index for assessment of molecular similarity. Croat Chem Acta 1993; 66:123-7.

211. Pepperrell CA, Willett P. Calculation of three-dimensional structural similarity. Chem Struct 1993; 2:377-82.

212. Richards WG. Molecular similarity. In: Wermuth C-G, ed. Trends in QSAR and Molecular Modelling 92. Leiden: ESCOM, 1993:203-6.

213. Randic M, Razinger M. Molecular topographic indices. J Chem Inf Comput Sci 1995; 35:140-7.

214. Good AC, Richards WG. Rapid evaluation of shape similarity using Gaussian functions. J Chem Inf Comput Sci 1993; 33:112-16.

215. Stanton DT, Murray WJ, Jurs PC. Comparison of QSAR and molecular similarity approaches for a structure-activity relationship study of DHFR inhibitors. Quant Struct Act Relat 1993; 12:239-45.

216. Seri-Levy A, West S, Richards WG. Molecular similarity, quantitative chirality, and QSAR for chiral drugs. J Med Chem 1994; 37:1727-32.

217. Seri-Levy A, Salter R, West S et al. Shape similarity as a single independent variable in QSAR. Eur J Med Chem 1994; 29:687-94.

218. Benigni R, Cotta-Ramusino M, Giorgi F et al. Molecular similarity matrixes and quantitative structure-activity relationships: a case study with methodological implications. J Med Chem 1995; 38:629-35.

219. Viswanadhan VN, Ghose AK, Revankar GR et al. Atomic physicochemical parameters for three dimensional structure directed quantitative structure-activity relationships. 4. Additional parameters for hydrophobic and dispersive interactions and their application for an automated superposition of certain naturally occurring nucleoside antibiotics. J Chem Inf Comput Sci 1989; 29:163-72.

220. Doweyko AM. The hypothetical active site lattice. An approach to modelling active sites from data on inhibitor molecules. J Med Chem 1988; 31:1396-406.

221. Doweyko AM. New tool for the study of structure-activity relationships in three dimensions. The hypothetical active-site lattice. Probing Bioactivity Mechanisms. Washington, DC: ACS, 1989: 82-104. ACS Symp. Ser; vol 413.

222. Wiese M. The hypothetical active-site lattice. In: Kubinyi H, ed. 3D QSAR in Drug Design: Theory Methods and Applications. Leiden: ESCOM, 1993:431-42.

223. Doweyko AM. Pharmacophores from binding data. J Med Chem 1994; 37:1769-78.

224. Saxena AK, Saxena M, Chi H et al. Identification of a pharmacophore by application of Hypothetical Active Site Lattice (HASL) approach. Med Chem Res 1993; 3:201-8.

225. Jain AN, Dietterich TG, Lathrop RH et al. Compass: a shape-based machine learning tool for drug design. J Comput-Aided Mol Des 1994; 8:635-52.

226. Jain AN, Harris NL, Park JY. Quantitative binding site model generation: Compass applied to multiple chemotypes targeting the 5-HT1A receptor. J Med Chem 1995; 38:1295-308.

227. Hahn M. Receptor surface models. 1. Definition and construction. J Med Chem 1995; 38:2080-90.

228. Rogers D, Hopfinger AJ. Application of genetic function approximation to quantitative structure-activity relationships and quantitative structure-property relationships. J Chem Inf Comput Sci 1994; 34:854-66.

229. Belvisi L, Bonati L, Bravi G et al. Structure-activity relationships of non-peptide angiotensin II antagonists. In: Wermuth C-G, ed. Trends in QSAR and Molecular Modelling 92. Leiden: ESCOM, 1993:312-13.

230. Belvisi L, Bravi G, Scolastico C et al. A 3D QSAR approach to the search for geometrical similarity in a series of nonpeptide angiotensin II receptor antagonists. J Comput-Aided Mol Des 1994; 8:211-20.

231. Pitea D, Cosentino U, Moro G et al. 3D QSAR: the integration of QSAR with molecular modeling. In: van de Waterbeemd H, ed. Advanced Computer-Assisted Techniques in Drug Discovery. Weinheim: VCH, 1995:9-38. (Mannhold R, Krogsgaard-Larsen P, Timmerman H, eds. Methods and Principles of Medicinal Chemistry; vol 3).

232. de Benedetti PG, Cocchi M, Menziani MC et al. Theoretical quantitative structure-activity analysis and pharmacophore modeling of selective non-congeneric α1a-adrenergic antagonists. Theochem 1993; 99:283-90.

233. Fanelli F, Menziani MC, Carotti A et al. Theoretical quantitative structure-activity relationship analysis on three dimensional models of ligand-m1 muscarinic receptor complexes. Bioorg Med Chem 1994; 2:195-211.

234. Fanelli F, Menziani MC, Cocchi M et al. The heuristic-direct approach to theoretical quantitative structure-activity relationship analysis of α1-adrenoceptor ligands. Theochem 1994; 120:265-76.

235. Mager PP. A2 agonists: structure-activity relationships of 2-(cycloalkylalkynyl)adenosine derivatives. Eur J Med Chem 1994; 29:369-80.

236. Mager PP. Multivariate analysis of cartesian coordinates of bioorganic molecules. In: Kuchar M, ed. QSAR in the Design of Bioactive. Compounds. Barcelona: Prous, 1992:446-69.

237. Holloway MK, Wai JM, Halgren TA et al. A priori prediction of activity for HIV-1 protease inhibitors employing energy minimization in the active site. J Med Chem 1995; 38:305-17.

238. Ortiz AR, Pisabarro MT, Gago F et al. Prediction of drug binding affinities by comparative binding energy analysis. J Med Chem 1995; 38:2681-91.

239. Golender VE, Vorpagel ER. Computer-assisted pharmacophore identification. In: Kubinyi H, ed. 3D QSAR in Drug Design: Theory Methods and Applications. Leiden: ESCOM, 1993:137-49.

240. APEX-3D. BIOSYM Technologies, Inc. San Diego, CA.

241. PRO_LIGAND. Proteus Molecular Design, Ltd. Macclesfield, UK.

242. CATALYST. Molecular Simulations, Inc. Burlington, NH.

243. Teig SL. The development of meaningful 3-D search queries for drug discovery. Recent Advances in Chemical Information II. 1993:195-208. Special Publ R Soc Chem; vol 120).

244. Itai A, Tomioka N, Yamada M et al. Molecular superposition for rational drug design. In: Kubinyi H, ed. 3D QSAR in Drug Design: Theory Methods and Applications. 1993:200-25.

245. Itai A, Tomioka N, Kato Y et al. New rational approaches for structure-activity relationships and drug design. In: Wermuth CG, ed. Medicinal Chemistry for the 21st Century. Oxford: Blackwell Scientific Publications, 1992:191-212.

246. Martin YC, Kim KH, Bures MG. Computer-assisted drug design in the 21st century. In: Wermuth CG, ed. Medicinal Chemistry for the 21st Century. Oxford: Blackwell Scientific Publications, 1992:295-317.

247. Klebe G. Structural alignment of molecules. In: Kubinyi H, ed. 3D QSAR in Drug Design: Theory Methods and Applications. Leiden: ESCOM, 1993:173-99.

248. Apaya RP, Lucchese B, Price SL et al. The matching of electrostatic extrema: A useful method in drug design? A study of phosphodiesterase III inhibitors. J Comput-Aided Drug Design 1995; 9:33-43.

249. Vinter JG. Extended electron distributions applied to the molecular mechanics of some intermolecular interactions. J Comput-Aided Mol Des 1994; 8:653-68.

250. Walters DE, Hinds RM. Genetically evolved receptor models: a computational approach to construction of receptor models. J Med Chem 1994; 37:2527-36.

251. Vinter GG, Trollope KI. Multiconformational composite molecular potential fields in the analysis of drug action. I. Methodology

and first evaluation using 5-HT and histamine action as examples. J Comp-Aided Mol Des 1995; 9:297-307.

252. Clark M, Cramer RD, III, Jones DM et al. Comparative molecular field analysis (CoMFA). 2. Toward its use with 3D-structural databases. Tetrahedron Comput Methodol 1990; 3:47-59.

253. Boehm H-J. The development of a simple empirical scoring function to estimate the binding constant for a protein-ligand complex of known three-dimensional structure. J Comput-Aided Mol Des 1994; 8:243-56.

254. Meng EC, Shoichet BK, Kuntz ID. Automated docking with grid-based energy evaluation. J Comput Chem 1992; 13:505-24.

255. Meng EC, Kuntz ID, Abraham DJ et al. Evaluating docked complexes with the HINT exponential function and empirical atomic hydrophobicities. J Comput Aided Mol Des 1994; 8:299-306.

256. Shoichet BK, Kuntz ID. Matching chemistry and shape in molecular docking. Protein Eng 1993; 6:723-32.

257. Lin CT, Pavlik PA, Martin YC. Use of molecular fields to compare series of potentially bioactive molecules designed by scientists or by computer. Tetrahedron Comput Methodol 1990; 3:723-38.

258. Martin YC, Bures MG, Danaher EA et al. The 3D design and potency forecast of biologically active molecules. In: Doyama M, ed. Computer Aided Innovation in New Materials, Vol. 2. Amsterdam: North-Holland, 1993:1117-20.

CHAPTER 6

APPLICATIONS OF MOLECULAR SIMILARITY/DISSIMILARITY IN DRUG RESEARCH

Michael S. Lajiness

Molecular similarity is a way to describe the relatedness between pairs of molecules in a nonspecific way. There are many ways that one can define molecular similarity and many ways to utilize this information in a pharmaceutical context. Much has been written about the use of similarity in drug research in the past several years. But what is it? How do we define it? And how can we use it to perform useful tasks? This chapter will attempt to provide answers to these questions based on experiences gained at The Upjohn Company since molecular similarity was first introduced in 1987.

The basis for computing the similarity between molecules lies in the representation scheme used and the method of computing the actual similarity value. Different methods will, of course, generate different values. Given a particular definition of similarity, for example, one can say that the benzodiazepines alprazolam and triazolam, appearing in Figure 6.1, are similar to each other by a value of 0.977.

Structure-Property Correlations in Drug Research, edited by Han van de Waterbeemd. © 1996 R.G. Landes Company.

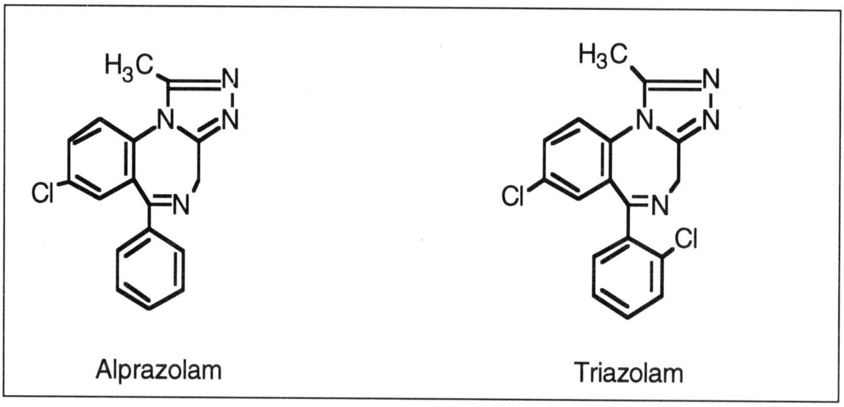

Fig. 6.1. Structures for the triazolo-benzodiazepines, alprazolam and triazolam.

On the other hand, using another definition, one could say that the Euclidean distance between these two compounds is 0.579. Which is right? Which definition should be used? These are actually difficult if not impossible, questions to answer. Since no two people will agree on the relative beauty of a sunset, can we expect things to be any different with respect to molecules? In addition, how will we judge the adequacy of the similarity value? Shall we use biological activity, melting point or clog P? The point here is that the calculated similarity value depends upon the similarity representation chosen and the method used to compute the similarity value. In addition, the choice of method will hinge on practical considerations such as ease of computation or accessibility. It is important to note that any resultant correlation with particular properties will depend on those choices!

In this chapter we will examine various methods of defining molecular similarity, how to use this information to diversify a given compound collection, select compounds for screening, and construct structurally diverse combinatorial libraries.

DEFINING MOLECULAR SIMILARITY

For an excellent introduction to similarity in chemistry the reader is referred to the first two chapters in the book "Concepts and Applications of Molecular Similarity."[1] Also, the landmark book by Peter Willett, *Similarity and Clustering in Chemical Information Systems*[2] provides an in depth evaluation and comparison of differ-

Table 6.1. Different methods to describe molecular similarity

2D
  Molecular fragments
  Topological/Information theoretic indices
  Atom pairs
  Chemical graphs
3D
  Molecular surfaces
  Steric volumes
  Electron densities
  Field potentials
  3D atomic configuration

Property-based
  Molecular property-based

ent structural representation schemes and corresponding calculation of similarity values.

Table 6.1 contains several methods that have been used to describe molecular similarity. The computational requirements necessary to define and utilize 3D-based similarity methods make them generally impractical in large database applications at the present time. This will, of course, change as computing power increases and more efficient methods are developed. Consequently, the focus of this chapter will be placed on 2D methods. In particular, we will focus on the methods that, in the authors opinion, are the most widely used today, namely similarity based on molecular fragments, and methods based on topological/information theoretic indices.

MOLECULAR FRAGMENT-BASED METHODS

Fragment-based methods generally utilize a bit vector, that is, a sequence of 0s and 1s that corresponds to the absence or presence of particular substructural features. A simple implementation of this sort of representation scheme for two compounds is illustrated in Figure 6.2. In this example, each bit corresponds to a single fragment. These fragment bits were originally created for efficient substructure searching before their use in a similarity context was conceived. The reader should note that this representation scheme is ambiguous since two different molecules *could* have the same representation although in practice this is of minimal concern. One should also note that in most implementations no account is made for the *number* of occurrences of each fragment and one cannot generally distinguish between stereoisomers.

The most popular way to compute the similarity between two molecules is by using the Tanimoto coefficient (TC) although other ways, such as Euclidean distance, have also been used. The TC is computed as follows:

$$TC = \frac{NC}{NC+ND}$$

where, NC = number of bits in common, and ND = number of bits that are different. The value of TC ranges between 0 (least similarity) and 1 (greatest similarity). If we computed the TC for the two compounds in Figure 6.2 using just the first 7 bits we would have the following results:

NC (number of bits in common)   = 3
ND (number of bits that are different)   = 1
TC (Tanimoto coefficient)   = 3/(3+1) = 3/4 = 0.75
Thus, the similarity between these two compounds is 0.75.

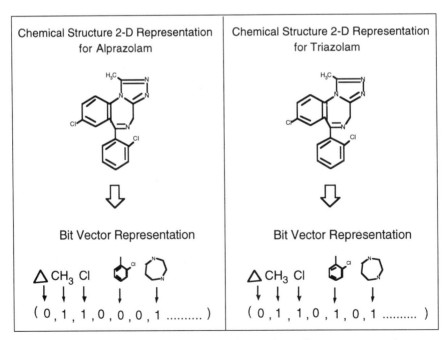

Fig. 6.2. Illustration of a fragment-bit representation scheme for two compounds.

This approach has been widely used and promulgated by Peter Willett and coworkers.[2,3] It should be noted that fragment bits are available for many of the popular chemical database systems such as Daylight and MACCS/ISIS software.

TOPOLOGICAL/INFORMATION THEORETIC INDICES

Another way to describe molecules is by examining the way atoms are connected in a molecule and the overall complexity of a molecule. Much work has been reported on the use of *"connectivity indices"* as well as on *"information theoretic indices"* which use calculations performed on the distance or adjacency matrix. An illustration of a distance and adjacency matrix can be found in Figure 6.3.

As can be seen in Figure 6.3 the symmetric adjacency and distance matrices are based on the hydrogen-suppressed graph, with each atom being arbitrarily numbered. The adjacency matrix is then formed by inserting a "1" into matrix element (i,j) if atom i is directly bonded to atom j. In the example above, atom $1(C_1)$ is directly attached to atom $2(C_2)$ so the (1,2) element in the adjacency matrix is "1." Similarly atom $2(C_2)$ is directly attached to atom $1(C_1)$, atom 3(N), and to atom 4(O). Thus, elements (2,1), (2,3), and (2,4) are all "1." Elements in the distance matrix reflect the number of bonds that separate atoms. So, if atom 1 is directly attached to atom 2 then element (1,2) is 1. Since atom 1 is 2 bonds away from atom 3, element (1,3) is 2. In the above example,

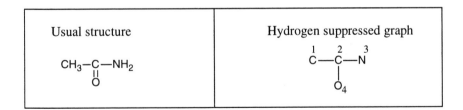

Usual structure	Hydrogen suppressed graph
CH_3-C-NH_2 ‖ O	1　2　3 C—C—N 	 O_4

Adjacency matrix

```
0 1 0 0
1 0 1 1
0 1 0 0
0 1 0 0
```

Distance matrix

```
0 1 2 2
1 0 1 1
2 1 0 2
2 1 2 0
```

Fig. 6.3. Example of an adjacency and distance matrix.

atom $1(C_1)$ is 1 bond away from atom $2(C_2)$ and 2 bonds away from atoms $3(N)$ and $4(O)$.

Two examples of topological/information theoretic indices that are used in similarity calculations are the Wiener Index (W) and the zero-order χ index ($^0\chi$). The W index is based on the distance matrix and is illustrated in Figure 6.4 below.

The $^0\chi$ index, on the other hand, is based on the adjacency matrix and is illustrated in Figure 6.5.

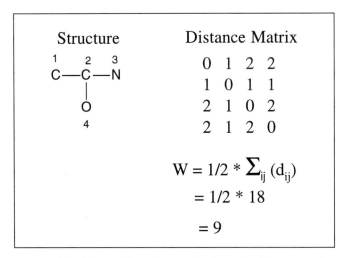

Fig. 6.4. Calculation of the Wiener Index from the distance matrix.

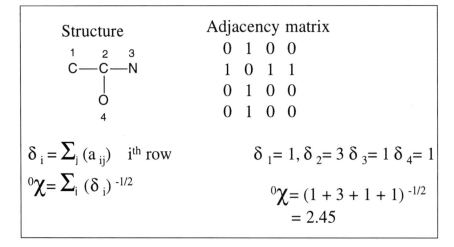

Fig. 6.5. Calculation of the $^0\chi$ index based on the adjacency matrix.

There are over one hundred topological/information theoretic indices that have been used in a chemistry context, relating structure to function. One worker in the field, S. Basak,[4] has developed an approach that condenses the information from many indices into a few by a dimension reduction technique called principal components analysis (PCA), and then uses Euclidean distance to measure the similarity between molecules. The technique consists of first calculating 96 indices for each of the n-molecules, log transforming the data (to remove the effect of outliers), performing a PCA on the n by 96 data matrix (to select the m-components that explain about 90% of the variance), and then standardizing the m-scores to a Standard Normal (N(0,1) distribution). The basic idea of the Basak approach is that by combining a multitude of different indices that have found utility in different applications, one can come up with a *global* similarity measure that has relevance in a variety of situations. This technique has been used successfully at Glaxo-Wellcome, and at The Upjohn Co.

OTHER TECHNIQUES

The Atom-Pair approach of Carhart et al[5] has been used successfully although it is not as widely used as the fragment and topological approaches. Molecular property-based similarity[6] has been implemented at Chemical Abstracts Service and appears to be a useful tool. Using chemical graphs per se and some of the ideas of graph theory to construct reasonable similarity applications on large databases is computationally unfeasible at the present time although some progress has been made to make the calculations more tractable.[7]

USE OF SIMILARITY INFORMATION IN DRUG RESEARCH

Molecular similarity has had a great impact on drug discovery research. The use of similarity in Drug Research primarily falls into two categories: similarity searching applications and dissimilarity selection applications. These will be discussed and illustrated below.

SIMILARITY SEARCHING

Similarity searching is a method to identify a set of compounds that are structurally related to a specified target molecule. In a drug research context, when an active compound is discovered in a biological assay one might use similarity searching to find related compounds to test. The essential idea here is that these compounds will have a higher than normal chance of being active. The guiding principal here is that *in general* similar compounds will elicit similar biological effects. Using one or more similarity searching methods (based on different representation schemes for example), one can explore the structure-activity surface in a region of chemical space that contains active compounds.

Similarity searching is available at The Upjohn Co. through the Cousin system,[8] an in-house developed chemical/biological information system. Currently, three methods are available to users: a fragment-based method utilizing 367 screening bits;[9] a modified-topological/information theoretic method based on the method of Basak;[4] and a maximum common subgraph method.[7] Typically, a variety of default parameters affecting the performance of the various similarity search methodologies are set. For example, for the fragment-based similarity method (using the Tanimoto coefficient) one can define:

1. the minimum similarity required (default = 0.67)
2. the maximum number of hits allowed (default = 50)
3. the target structure (via custom drawing or reference code)

By adjustment of these parameters you can tune the searches to meet your own needs.

Figures 6.6 and 6.7 present some results of similarity searches on the ACD database using a fragment-based search for compounds related to aspirin.

DISSIMILARITY SELECTION

Dissimilarity selection is a method whereby one selects compounds that are structurally different from one another. In a pharmaceutical context one might use dissimilarity selection to identify a set of structurally diverse compounds to screen first in a selected biological assay. The idea here is that if similar compounds cause similar biological effects, different or diverse structures should produce different effects. Thus, by looking at diverse structures in an assay one can rapidly identify those regions of chemical space that contain active compounds. One can then use similarity searching to further explore structure-activity relationships as discussed above.

There are a variety of ways that one can choose dissimilar sets of molecules once a representation in a similarity space is made. D-optimal designs have been used[10] as well as cluster analysis,[2,11-13]

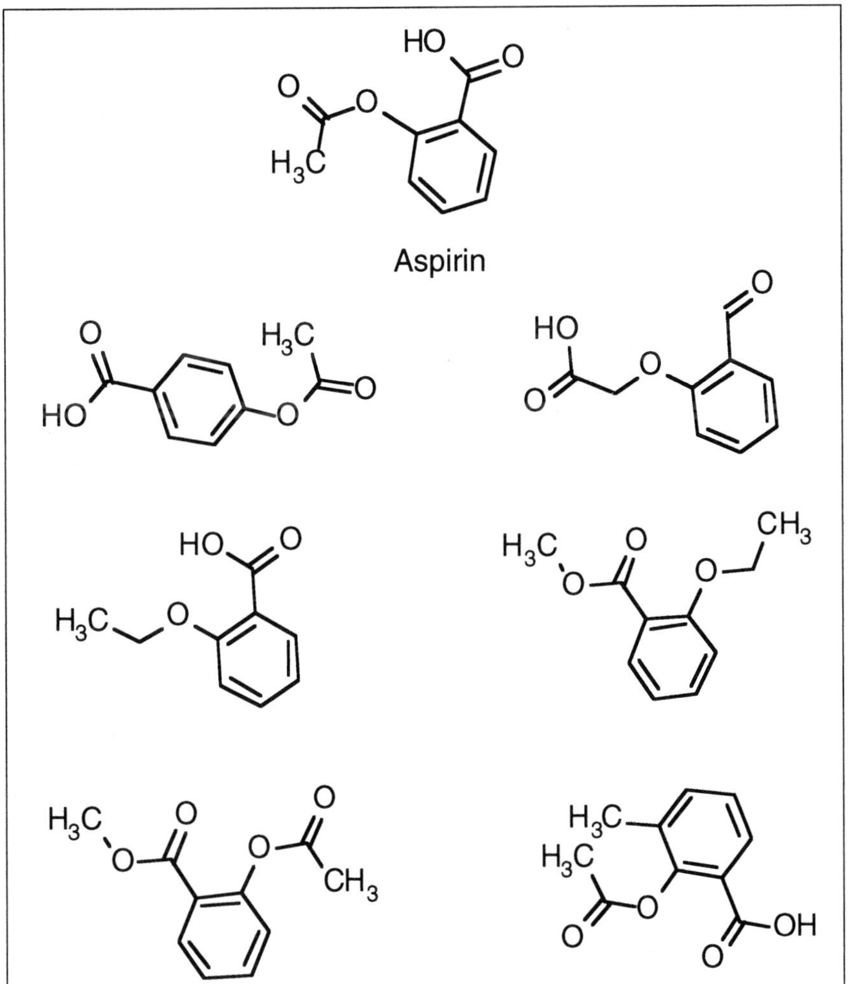

Fig. 6.6. Six compounds from the ACD that are similar to aspirin using a fragment-based representation.

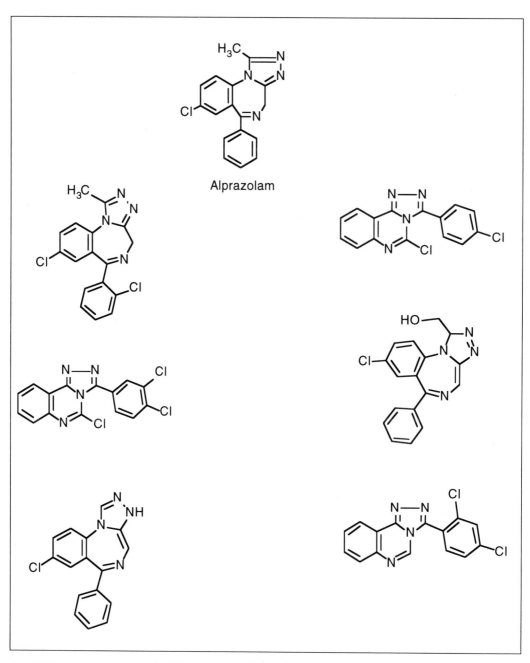

Fig. 6.7. Six compounds from the ACD that are similar to alprazolam using a fragment-based representation.

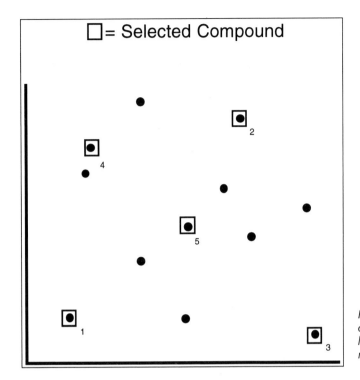

Fig. 6.8. Illustration of dissimilarity selection by the MD method.

and maximum dissimilarity selection.[9,14-17] Figure 6.8 illustrates the maximum dissimilarity (MD) selection method which has been used at Upjohn since 1987. In the MD method, a compound is picked randomly (indicated by a box with a subscripted one) and then a calculation is made to determine the compound that is furthest from it in terms of dissimilarity. If one is dealing with a fragment-based representation one can use (1-TC), where TC is the value of the Tanimoto coefficient discussed previously, to define what is meant by dissimilarity. This dissimilarity metric would then range from 1 (highest dissimilarity) to 0 (lowest dissimilarity).

As mentioned previously, cluster analysis can also be used to select dissimilar sets of compounds. In this method, illustrated in Figure 6.9, compounds are clustered together using a non-hierarchical clustering procedure (such as the SAS Procedure FASTCLUS[18]). Nonhierarchical clustering generally requires the specification of the number of clusters to be generated. This is usually taken to be the number of compounds desired to be selected. If, for example, five structurally diverse compounds are desired to be chosen from 12, then one would generate 5 clusters as seen in Figure 6.9. Once the clustering is accomplished, one compound needs to be selected from each cluster to obtain the requisite number. The compound nearest the cluster center (centroid) is usually used for this purpose.

Pseudocode to perform the dissimilarity selection can be found in Table 6.2.

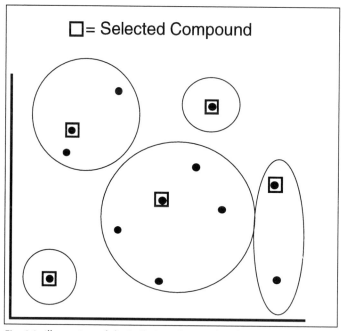

Fig. 6.9. Illustration of dissimilarity selection by clustering.

Table 6.2. Maximum dissimilarity program description

- Choose dissimilarity descriptor (e.g. 1-TC)
- Create comparison vector of size n of 1s (1,1,1....1)
    (n is the number of compounds)
- Choose a compound randomly
- Zero its entry in comparison vector
- Calculate dissimilarities to chosen compounds
- If dissimilarity value for compound i is less than corresponding vector value
    then replace entry with calculated dissimilarity
- After all compounds are processed, find index corresponding to largest
    element in vector; call it j
- Choose compound j (assuming uniqueness)
- Repeat steps 4-7 until number of compounds desired is selected

SELECTING DIVERSE COMPOUNDS FOR SCREENING

Dissimilarity selection technology was first developed and used at Upjohn in 1987 and has been described earlier in this chapter. The problem of selecting diverse compounds for screening can be divided into two cases: when no compounds have been screened; and, when compounds have been screened already. In the case when one wishes to select diverse compounds when no screening has yet occurred, we basically have the case of "normal" dissimilarity selection as discussed in the previous section (Table 6.2). That is, we start with a set of available compounds and choose the most diverse compounds based on the MD method for example. The set of "available" compounds being those compounds that meet a set of predefined criteria such as having sufficient inventory available for testing, structures that contain at least one nitrogen atom, no steroids or prostaglandins, etc. In the case where compounds have already been screened, the problem is slightly different. The problem now is to choose a set of compounds that are structurally different than the compounds already screened. An illustration of the MD method applied to this problem can be found in Figure 6.10. To choose the first compound, one calculates which of the available compounds are furthest (most dissimilar) to any compound already screened (indicated by a square and a subscripted one in the figure). Subsequent compounds are selected in a similar manner to be dissimilar from compounds already tested as well as those already selected.

The factors affecting the performance of cluster-based(CB) and maximum dissimilarity (MD) selection methods versus random selection has been investigated previously.[14] Simulation experiments were conducted examining how changes in the distribution of active compounds in the chemical descriptor space affect the ability to select compounds from unique clusters of active compounds. It was found that the distribution of active compounds does affect the performance of dissimilarity selection. The MD method was shown to be most effective in locating the active clusters. In addition, the performance of the methods was compared in a retrospective experiment using anthelmintic data. In this experiment, the three methods, Random, CB, and MD selection, were used to select compounds from the set already screened for anthelmintic

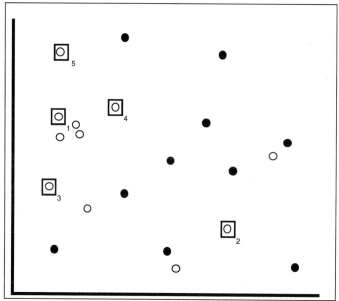

☐ = Selected Compound

● =Already screened compound

○ =Compound available for screening

Fig. 6.10. Illustration of dissimilarity selection when compounds have already been screened.

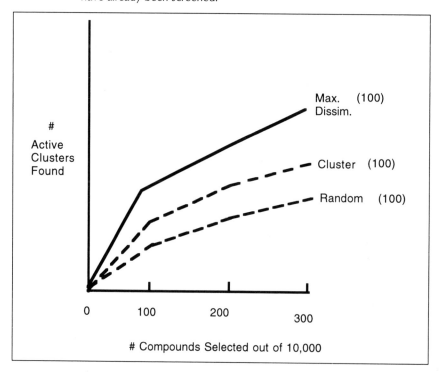

Fig. 6.11. Empirical performance of dissimilarity and cluster-based selection.

activity. Once selected, their biological activity was determined from the historical record and the number of "unique active clusters" counted. Each method was repeated 100 times and averages calculated. The results, summarized in Figure 6.11, indicated that the MD method was about 1.5 to 2.0 times more effective than random selection and about 1.3 to 1.4 times more effective than cluster-based selection in terms of finding active clusters of compounds.

SELECTING COMPOUNDS FOR PURCHASE

There has been much recent interest in the topic of combinatorial chemistry and the potential amount of structural diversity that can be generated by such collections. There is another source of readily available compounds that contain even more structural diversity, namely, commercially available compounds from suppliers such as Aldrich and Sigma. While for many years many companies have routinely acquired compounds to augment their proprietary compound collections, it is only recently that computer programs have been designed to select pharmaceutically relevant compounds from the ACD that are structurally diverse and different from compounds already contained in the proprietary database. The following will describe a methodology developed at The Upjohn Company to systematically diversify its compound database by strategic purchase of selected compounds from the ACD. This involved the development of a computer-assisted process based on molecular dissimilarity techniques to select compounds from commercially available databases that were structurally most dissimilar to those compounds currently in the Upjohn compound database. Numerous exclusion criteria based on medicinal chemists' suggestions were used to eliminate compounds considered unsuitable as potential lead structures. The resultant list of compounds is then used as a basis for purchase recommendations allowing the construction of a structurally diverse database of compounds in a rapid and efficient manner.

INTRODUCTION

The existence of a structurally diverse compound repository is essential to the rapid discovery of novel lead compounds. But where will these compounds come from and how can one identify that set of molecules that would best suit the particular compound collection? It was decided to develop a computer-based procedure to assist in the identification of compounds that were most structurally different from compounds in our proprietary collection. This is necessary since the size of the collections involved are much too great to expect humans to perform the task.

A prerequisite for construction of such a process was the availability of *computer searchable databases of structures for purchase.* Currently included as part of the Cousin System[8] are two databases containing candidate compounds for purchase: the Available Chemicals Directory (ACD); and the Commercial Research Compounds Directory (CRCD). These databases together contain over 300,000 compounds.

Given a fairly large supply of candidate molecules it is necessary to identify a relatively small number that might make reasonable additions to the Upjohn proprietary collection. In pursuit of this goal, software was developed to identify structures from external sources (namely the ACD and CRCD) that were maximally different from compounds already in the repository. This "Dissimilarity Selection" software utilizes fragment-bit string structure representations that are used as part of the Cousin substructure searching and similarity searching systems.

It soon became apparent that not all compounds in the available databases would be reasonable choices in a pharmaceutical context. Thus, it was desired that the lists of recommended compounds not include those structures generally considered unsuitable as lead compounds. This prompted the development of *exclusion criteria* that allowed us to focus our activities on compounds that were most appropriate for lead finding purposes.

There are several steps and issues involved in the process of compound selection. The remainder of this section will be devoted to the further elucidation of the procedure and documentation of the methodology used.

ACCESSING CANDIDATE COMPOUND LIBRARIES

Many suppliers of compounds provide electronic versions of their databases that can be incorporated into Cousin. These have

Table 6.3. List of CRCD Suppliers

Aldrich
Bader/Rare Chem Lib
Bionet Research Ltd.
Bob Harmon, WMU
Brandon Specs
ComGenex
Dr. Alan Katritzky
Dr. Bernard Blessington
Dr. Nash (Wye College)
Labotest
Maybridge (Ryan)
Menai Organics
Merlin Synthesis
Peakdale Fine Chemicals
SZS Technologies

been divided into separate databases in Cousin. The ACD corresponds to major commercial sources of compounds where one can count on the compounds being available (e.g., Aldrich, Sigma, etc). It currently includes about 185,000 compounds. The CRCD, on the other hand, consists typically of smaller vendors of compounds where the supply of compound may be small or nonexistent (for example, university-based sources such as Dr. Katritzky at Univ. of Florida, Gainesville). The CRCD currently includes about 250,000 compounds. Some of the suppliers available in the CRCD are listed in Table 6.3.

FORMATION OF THE EXCLUSION SET

Review of initial lists of maximally dissimilar structures identified the presence of numerous compounds considered unsuitable for a variety of reasons (e.g., stability concerns). Several experienced medicinal chemists were then asked to identify the structural "themes" to remove the majority of the unsuitable compounds. This has resulted in the formation of a set of exclusion criteria (Figs. 6.12-6.14) that is used to filter prospective compounds. Cousin-based substructure searching along with general Cousin commands are used to form this exclusion set.

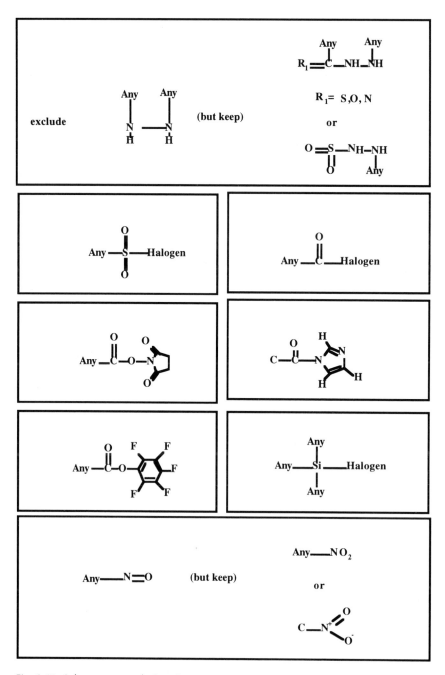

Fig. 6.12. Substructure exclusions I.

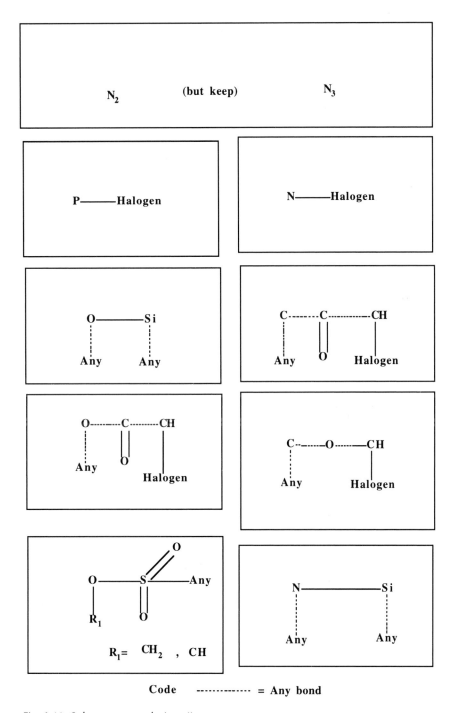

Fig. 6.13. Substructure exclusions II.

I. Undesired Transition Metals: Sc, Ti, V, Cr, Mn, Fe, Co,
                                   Ni, Cu, Zn,Ga,Ge,As

●

II. Undesired Transition Metals: Y, Zr, Nb, Mo, Tc, Ru,
                                   Rh, Pd, Ag, Cd

●

Misc. Undesired Elements: Be,B,Sn,Sb,Te,Ce,Tb,W,
                                   Re,Ir,Pt,Hg, Pb

●

Molecular weights of less than 100 or greater than 1,000.

●

Total number of Carbon atoms less than or equal to 4.

●

Compounds without a N, O, or S.

Fig. 6.14. Miscellaneous exclusion criteria.

DISSIMILARITY SELECTION

Once unsuitable compounds have been removed, the selection of compounds that are maximally different from those already in the proprietary database can proceed. Software to perform the *dissimilarity selection* was developed at Upjohn and runs on an IBM 3090 series 400. The methodology to perform dissimilarity selection at Upjohn as well as some of the results from using the methodology have been previously described. It should be noted that the computational resources required for dissimilarity selection may be considerable, and depend on the size of the databases concerned. For example, selection of 5,000 compounds from a set of 200,000 commercially available compounds most dissimilar to 100,000 Upjohn compounds takes about three weeks of computer time.

MEDICINAL CHEMISTRY REVIEW

Once a diverse collection of compounds has been identified, the structures are printed out and reviewed by medicinal chemistry staff. Compounds that, for a variety of reasons, are unsuitable are eliminated at this stage (typically less than 1%). This step may also point out new exclusion criteria that can then be defined and integrated into the process described above.

OTHER ISSUES

Selecting compounds from databases such as the ACD, which contain many suppliers, can present ordering logistical problems. We've addressed this by focusing on certain suppliers (based on volume, ease of interaction, etc) and limiting our attention to them. Registering compounds upon receipt was a headache until a "batch" process was implemented in the Cousin System—another advantage to having our "own" chemical/biology database system. Sample preparation was made easier by working directly with suppliers to provide compatible sample vials. One issue we have not dealt with effectively so far is that of price versus dissimilarity. The cost of many compounds is not currently available to us electronically, which we hope will be remedied in the near future.

SUMMARY AND CONCLUSIONS

Increasing the structural diversity of proprietary databases has increased the likelihood of discovering important new lead compounds. The availability of an integrated and flexible chemical/biological information system is essential to the database augmentation process, and Cousin provides us with a very good one. Cousin-based dissimilarity selection programs, in conjunction with standard database operations such as substructure searching, can form the basis for rational compound selection practices that can have a big impact on the success of a lead discovery program.

EVALUATING THE DIVERSITY OF COLLECTIONS OF COMPOUNDS

Another approach to increasing the diversity of compounds subject to biological screening efforts is through the combinatorial chemistry-type programs. But how does one evaluate the relative diversity of different combinatorial chemistry approaches? What types of diversity measurements are relevant? Is diversity an absolute, or is it relative?

Before we consider the answers to the questions posed above, consider the following example illustrated in Figure 6.15. Let's assume that a company's available chemical inventory (the proprietary collection) occupies a certain region of a chemical descriptor space, as represented by graph (i) in Figure 6.15. Also, assume that there are two combinatorial libraries (graphs ii and iii) that are offered to the company to enhance the diversity of their proprietary collection. (Call these libraries, Library 1 and Library 2.) Notice that these two libraries occupy about the same *volume* of space in the illustration and can be considered as equally diverse relative to the total chemical descriptor space. However, if one considers the diversity of Library 1 and Library 2 relative to the proprietary collection, (graphs iv and v), it is clear that Library 2 would enhance the diversity of the company collection the most. This example is intended to emphasize the point that diversity is not necessarily an absolute. Therefore, the relevant calculation that needs to be made when evaluating combinatorial library approaches is the amount of structural diversity contained in the proposed libraries *relative* to the proprietary collection. The remainder of this section will describe a way to evaluate the relative diversity of collections of compounds using molecular similarity and dissimilarity ideas in conjunction with standard statistical techniques.

The technique about to be described assumes the existence of a suitable structural representation scheme such as the fragment bits described earlier. Thus, to compare the relative diversity of two combinatorial libraries one needs to generate the appropriate structural descriptors for all compounds to be contained in these libraries. Many of the chemical database software providers are now able to generate these descriptors.

To illustrate a method for comparing the relative structural diversity between two collections of compounds, sets of prepared microtiter plates were chosen. These sets of prepared plates have been offered by commercial suppliers and supposedly contain diverse collections of compounds. Due to a nondisclosure requirement, the three collections used will be referred to as platesets I,

II, and III. Thus, the problem we wish to address is which of the platesets offer the greatest diversity relative to the Upjohn Collection.

Once similarity descriptors (i.e. fragment bits) have been generated for the compounds of interest one can compute the "dissimilarity" between each compound in a given plateset versus compounds in the Upjohn database. These calculations are exactly the same type as described earlier in the "Selecting Diverse Compounds

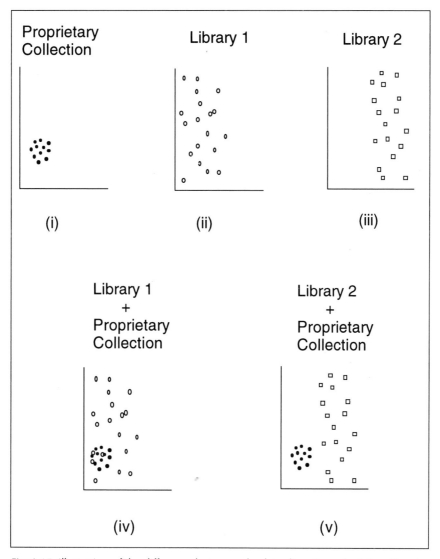

Fig. 6.15. Illustration of the difference between absolute diversity and relative diversity.

for Screening" section. Thus, for platesets I, for example, dissimilarities are computed for each compound. This dissimilarity represents the "distance" a compound is relative to the "nearest" compound in the Upjohn collection or to a compound from plateset I that has already been "selected." So, each dissimilarity run produces a set of dissimilarities that form a distribution that can be analyzed using statistical techniques. One way to analyze distributions is the boxplot, which is available in SAS Software through the Univariate procedure.[18] Histograms and corresponding boxplots illustrating the distributions of dissimilarities for each plateset appear in Figure 6.16.

Please note that the boxplot summarizes the distribution of a set of data. For example, the bottom and top edges of the box are located at the sample 25th and 75th percentiles (the interquartile range). The center horizontal line is drawn at the sample median. The central vertical lines (wiskers) extend from the box as far as the data extend, to a distance of at most 1.5 interquartile ranges.

Examination of the distribution of dissimilarities displayed in Figure 6.16 indicates that plateset II appears to have the least dissimilarity to the Upjohn Collection, while platesets I and III were

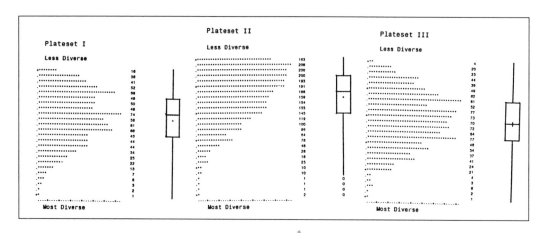

Fig. 6.16. Distribution of dissimilarities for platesets I, II, and III.

Quantile	Plateset I	Plateset II	Plateset III
10	.15	.05	.09
25	.24	.11	.17
50 (Median)	.37	.23	.30
75	.49	.36	.42
90	.60	.48	.52
99	.75	.67	.69
Mean	.37	.25	.31

Fig. 6.17. Sample quantiles for dissimilarity distributions.

fairly comparable. Looking at the sample quantile estimates in Figure 6.17, (also produced by the UNIVARIATE procedure), one can quantitatively evaluate the dissimilarities and conclude that purchase of plateset I would add the most diversity to the Upjohn proprietary collection. It should be pointed out that results *will* depend on the database upon which the comparison is based.

In summary, it appears that analysis of the distribution of dissimilarities can be a useful tool to determine the relative structural diversity of collections of compounds. This should, of course, apply to combinatorial libraries as well.

CONCLUDING REMARKS

There are many ways that one can utilize molecular similarity in drug research applications. Molecular similarity-based thinking should become even more useful with the advent of combinatorial chemistry and the interest placed on the structural diversity of compound data collections. The number of possible applications is only limited by our imaginations.

REFERENCES

1. Johnson MA, Maggiora GM, eds. Concept and Applications of Molecular Similarity. John Wiley, New York, 1990.

2. Willett P. Similarity and Clustering in Chemical Information Systems. Research Studies Press, 1987.

3. Willett P, Winterman VA. Comparison of some measures for the determination of inter-molecular structural similarity measures of inter-molecular structural similarity. Quant Struct-Act Relat 1986; 5:18-25.

4. Basak SC, Magnuson VR, Niemi GJ, Regal RR. Determining structural similarity of chemicals using graph-theoretic indices. Discrete Appl Math 1988; 19:17; Special Volume: Applications of Graph Theory in Chemistry and Physics, Kennedy JW, Quintas LV, eds.

5. Carhart RE, Smith DH, Venkataraghavan R. Atom pairs as molecular features in structure-activity studies: definition and application. J Chem Inform Comput Sci 1985; 25:64-73.

6. Fisanick W, Lipkus AH, Rusinko A. Similarity Searching on CAS Registry Substances. II. 2D Structural Similarity (in press).

7. Hagadone TR. Molecular substructure similarity searching: efficient retrieval in two-dimensional structure databases. J Chem Inform Comput Sci 1992; 32:515-21.

8. Hagadone TR, Lajiness MS. Capturing chemical information in an extended relational database system. Tetrahedron Comput Meth 1988; 1(3):219-30.

9. Lajiness MS. Molecular similarity-based method for selecting compounds for screening. In: Rouvray DH, ed. Computational Chemical Graph Theory. 1990: 299-316.

10. Martin EJ, Blaney JM, Siani MA, Spellmeyer DC, Wong AK, Moos WH. Measuring diversity: experimental design of combinatorial libraries for drug discovery. J Med Chem 1995; 38:1431-36.

11. Barnard JM, Down GM. J Chem Inf Comput Sci 1992; 32:644-649.

12. Willett P, Winterman V, Bawden D. J Chem Inf Comput Sci 1986; 26:109-18.

13. Hodes L. J Chem Inf Comput Sci 1989; 29:66-71.

14. Lajiness MS. An evaluation of the performance of dissimilarity selection. In: Silipo C, Vittoria A, eds. QSAR: Rational Approaches to the Design of Bioactive Compounds. Elsevier Science Publishers, Amsterdam, 1991:201-4.

15. Bawden D. Applications of two-dimensional chemical similarity measures to database analysis and querying. In: Johnson MA, Maggiora GM, eds. Concept and Applications of Molecular Similarity. John Wiley, New York, 1990:65-76.

16. Bawden D. Molecular dissimilarity in chemical information systems. In: Warr WA, ed. Chemical Structures 2. Springer Verlag, Heidelberg, 1993:383-8.
17. Lajiness MS Johnson MA, Maggiora GM. Implementing drug screening programs using molecular similarity methods. In: Fauchère JL, ed. QSAR: Quantitative Structure Activity Relationships in Drug Design, 1989:173-6.
18. SAS Institute Inc. SAS/STAT Users Guide, Version 6, Fourth Edition, 1989. Vol 1, Cary, NC: SAS Institute Inc.

INDEX

Items in italics denote figures (f) or tables (t).